MUSCLES AND MOVEMENTS

a basis for
human kinesiology

MUSCLES AND MOVEMENTS

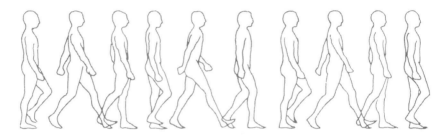

a basis for human kinesiology

M. A. MacConaill, M.A., M.B., D.Sc., M.R.I.A.

Professor of Anatomy
University College, Cork, Ireland

J. V. Basmajian, M.D.

Director of Research and Associate Director, Regional Rehabilitation
Research and Training Center, and Professor of Anatomy
Emory University, Atlanta, Georgia, U.S.A.

Formerly Head, Department of Anatomy
Queen's University, Kingston, Ontario, Canada

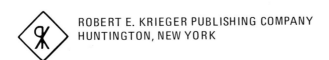
ROBERT E. KRIEGER PUBLISHING COMPANY
HUNTINGTON, NEW YORK

Original edition 1969
New Revised edition 1977

Printed and Published by
ROBERT E. KRIEGER PUBLISHING CO., INC.
645 NEW YORK AVENUE
HUNTINGTON, NEW YORK 11743

Library of Congress Cataloging in Publication Data

MacConaill, Michael Aloysius, 1902-
   Muscles and movements.

   Includes bibliographies and index.
   1. Kinesiology.   I. Basmajian, John V., 1921-
joint author.   II. Title.
QP303.M22   1976   612'.76   76-6883
ISBN 0-88275-398-3

Printed in the U.S.A. by
Noble Offset Printers Inc.
New York, N. Y. 10003

Preface to Second Edition

In preparing this edition we have been guided by the opinions of teachers and students on both sides of the Atlantic who have used the earlier book. Full note has been taken of both public and private criticisms of that text — our own included. As before, we have remembered that English is a foreign language to many of our readers, and we have tried to steer a middle course between over-idiomatic English and equally unintelligible Graeco-Latin jargon.

We have used some new words where these made for brevity and clarity. All of them are, of course, defined; and most of them have already appeared in our scientific publications.

The section on general muscle mechanics is now divided into two chapters, one on myokinematics, the other on myokinetics. This has been done in response to requests for a fuller treatment of both topics. The necessary mathematics has been kept at a simple level, matter for specialist readers being again put in the appendices. The two topics we have found to be linked by a common factor, the Partition-ratio, used in the earlier edition but not named until some years later. This double function of the ratio gives meaning to the otherwise tedious details of the origins and insertions of muscles — at least, that is how we found them to be when we were much younger students than we are now.

On one matter we have stood firm against some critics. We have retained the terms 'spurt' and 'shunt' in relation to muscular structure and function. Our reasons are given in the text. Those who would change them must find (or invent) other words equally simple and comprehensive in their scope. Meanwhile we are gratified with the increasing understanding of both the terms and their underlying concepts among clinicians and scientists.

Practical problems in preparing a new edition have been surprisingly small. The generous act of transferring the copyright to the authors by the publishers of the first edition (Williams & Wilkins Co.) permitted us to enlarge the work. We are grateful to John Krieger for the friendly cooperation that has marked our work together in this edition. We also thank Arlene De Bevoise for the excellent secretarial assistance without which our efforts would have been much less pleasant.

M.A. MacConaill

J.V. Basmajian

1976

Preface to First Edition

This book is what its title declares it to be: a study of bodily movements and of the muscles that bring them about. It is also what its subtitle declares it to be: a scientific basis for the subject, not a complete account of it. The reader will find in it something about the muscular forces that are involved in the statics and dynamics of the body. But we believe that much of what has been written on this topic is so speculative and based upon unverified hypotheses that it would be wrong for us to pretend to a knowledge that we do not possess. Bio-engineering is still an infant science. It is our hope that what we have written here may be of value to those who are helping this infant towards maturity.

Our book is intended as a complement to *Synovial Joints: Their Structure and Mechanics*, of which one of us was a co-author. Certain aspects of the physics of movement are dealt with more thoroughly here than was possible in the other work, in which mathematical treatment was kept to a very bare minimum. Mathematics is indispensable if kinesiology is to be more than a set of statements learnt by rote, if it is to be understood in such a way that it can both explain what we do know about movements and muscles and also form the basis of further, fruitful inquiry. We have included what is necessary but no more than is sufficient, allowing an orderly presentation of our main theses. As far as possible we have kept unfamiliar kinds of mathematics out of the text. However, that dealing with the general theory of the kinematics of bones and joints is of fundamental importance, and we have put it in an appendix for the convenience of those who wish to go more deeply into the subject.

This book also complements *Muscles Alive: Their Functions Revealed by Electromyography*; where information is derived from that larger and more specialized work, it has been modified extensively. Particular attention has been given to preparing new illustrations that present ideas rather than details.

There is one unavoidable deficiency in the pages that follow: incompleteness. While we were writing, while these pages were being printed, new additions were being made to our knowledge, particularly in the realm of electromyography. We make no apology for this deficiency; for all other faults we ask the reader's indulgence.

All 133 drawings for the present book are by one artist, Mr. Frank Edwards of Queen's University. For his intelligent conversion of our ideas and rough sketches into informative and elegant illustrations, we are truly grateful. Some of the figures are based on drawings in our earlier papers; we owe special thanks to the Royal Irish Academy for permission to reproduce or copy figures from its Proceedings. Our thanks also go to the many friends and colleagues from whom we have derived much useful information and continuing inspiration; the references in individual chapters give only a limited view of the scope of .this assistance. Finally, we thank our secretaries, Miss Finula O'Donovan and Mrs. Eleanor Teepell for their patience and care with the manuscript and Miss Mary Joan Deir and Mrs. Patricia Burt for their work on the index.

M.A. MacC.

J.V.B.

Alphabetic Symbols Used in Text

NOTE: Because of the shortness of the Latin alphabet and our reluctance to use the more unfamiliar Greek, some of the symbols are occasionally given different meanings from those defined below. Such uses are always stated clearly.

A: total angle of swing

a: speed of swing

B: angle between force-vector and a bone

b: speed of change of B

c: cisaxial length (of myoneme origin to swing-axis)

D: difference of A from $180°$

d: as in differential calculus (rarely used)

E: work done in raising gravicentre against gravity

e: work done by total musculature on bone

F: symbolizes a force

f: magnitude of a force

g: acceleration due to gravity (32 feet or 981 cm. per sec. per sec.)

h: vertical displacement of gravicentre by swing

i: initial angle between arc and chord in arcuate motion

j: total static transarticular force

k: kinetic energy of swinging bone

m: mass of a bone

n: Newtonian centripetal force (due to swing)

p: partition-ratio (c/q) of myoneme

q: transarticular length (of myoneme insertion to swing-axis)

R: angle of spin

r: length from swing-axis to gravicentre

ρ(rho):   the ratio r/q (radial ratio)

S: spurt-shunt ratio (myokinetics)

s: length of fully stretched myoneme (myokinematics); magnitude of spurt force (myokinetics)

t: proportion of tendon in a myoneme (myokinematics); magnitude of shunt force (myokinetics); terminal angle between chord and arc in arcuate motion

v: tangential velocity of swinging gravicentre

w: weight of bone (*plus* load carried by it)

x: "Undetermined multiplier" of $cos^2 A/2$ (myokinetics)

y: length of arcuate myoneme after it causes spin

z: length of totally contracted myoneme

Mathematical Signs Used in Text
(examples of use)

$x = y$: x is equal to (or equivalent to) y

$x > y$: x is greater than y

$x < y$: x is less than y

$x \geq y$:   *x is equal to or greater than y*

$x \leq y$: x is equal to or less than y

x / y: ratio of x to y

Contents

Part Three.   SPECIAL KINESIOLOGY

Part One
NATURE AND METHOD
OF KINESIOLOGY

ONE

"Kinesiology" means the study of movement, for us the study of movements of the bones and at the joints of the human body. It is a necessary part of all basic medical and dental training, as well as of the training of orthopaedic surgeons, specialists in physical medicine and such ancillary experts as physiotherapists, occupational therapists and physical education specialists. The study of movements must, however, be supported by a study of the means by which they are either brought about or restrained. These include gravity, the skeletal muscles and the mechanics of the joints. We take it for granted that the reader has such a knowledge of the anatomy of the locomotor system as is obtainable from the books listed at the end of this chapter. Our purpose is to help him or her to understand how structure is correlated with function in the living body, particularly in the light of modern knowledge. Such an understanding has always been desirable. Today, it has become increasingly essential; doctors and engineers are coöperating more and more, not only in assisting this understanding but also in applying it to the problems of daily life that affect the healthy as well as the sick.

As in all branches of knowledge, there are two kinds of kinesiology—basic and advanced. The advanced kinesiologist is one who combines the theoretical and practical skill of an engineer with the theoretical and practical skill of a medical scientist. Nowadays he is called a bio-engineer or, worse, a bio-medical engineer. He is an expert able to quarrel with, often to agree with, others of his lofty kind. These pages will not make their readers bio-engineers, but, to use an old English phrase, they may make the "makings" of bio-engineers. They are chiefly intended to let the present or future enquirer into human biology see how the movements of his body, things he knows very well, are brought about by the muscles and joints, things he knows less well.

All increase of knowledge is gained by someone doing something, somehow and somewhere. In other words, there is a *methodology* proper to every branch of science. Within one and the same science several methods of investigation become available as the science progresses. Indeed, progress depends upon there being more than one method, for each method helps to answer a different type of question, and the science itself consists of the fitting together of the correspondingly different types of information to form, if possible, a coherent and intellectually satisfying whole. This whole will never be quite coherent, quite satisfying. There is always more to find out, always some new application. Galileo, that highly intelligent (and highly irascible) Italian, pointed out that any hypothesis that seemed to cover everything was to be looked at suspiciously!

The aim of any methodology is to provide the material that will form the foundation of a science. Science itself has been defined as a knowledge of things by their causes; we recall the words of Horace, the Roman poet:

Felix qui potuit rerum cognoscere causas
(Happy is he who knoweth things by their causes).

Let us, then, take a look at the methodology of our subject, bodily motions and their causes.

METHODOLOGY

Kinesiology is a branch of physics, of mechanics in fact. It has three sources of knowledge: observation, experiment and theory. We shall examine each in turn and then consider their interrelations.

Observation

We can observe the movements of our own bones and those of others. This needs no further statement at the moment.

We can also examine muscles, bones and joints in the cadaver and draw some useful immediate inferences therefrom. For example, if we know the attachments (origin and insertion) of the brachialis muscle, *and* if we know that a muscle acts by pulling upon a bone, *and* if we know the movements permitted at the ulnohumeral joint, then we can infer that the brachialis *can* flex the ulnohumeral joint. Let us examine this simple instance further.

The thing is a piece of logic, like a theorem in Euclid's geometry: *if* certain things are true *then* a certain conclusion follows. Knowing the relevant structural facts about the brachialis, a functional fact about all muscles attached to bones and the functional facts about a joint on which the muscle acts, we infer that it can flex the said joint. But that is as far as observation takes us. Observation of the whole elbow joint shows us that the ulna may be flexed on the humerus by flexor muscles moving the radius; the biceps brachii is such a muscle. But observation is unable to tell which muscle or set of muscles of those of several that can flex the elbow actually do flex it in some given set of circumstances. In a word, observation alone tells us only the *functional potentialities* of this or that muscle, not its *functional acts*.

Experiment

There are two kinds of experiment upon muscles, visuo-tactile and electrical.

VISUO-TACTILE. This is simply a formal name for an old, old practice. We move some part of the body and try to ascertain what muscles are involved by looking and feeling. In particular, a given movement is carried out against resistance, and if some muscle is found to swell and harden or its tendon to become prominent, then it is inferred that this muscle is operative in the given movement. We shall consider the validity of this inference later. Meanwhile we note that it is sometimes possible to employ a simple visual test for determining when a muscle *relaxes*. A classic and easy example is furnished by the deltoid. Let a man abduct the shoulder so that the arm is horizontal. Place a weight upon the swollen deltoid. Then support the arm from below: the weight sinks downwards, showing that the deltoid has relaxed and ceased to operate.

ELECTRICAL (1). After Galvani had shown that an electric current could make a frog's muscle contract, it was natural that his experiment should be extended to man. The first to do this in a systematic way appears to have been Duchenne (1867), who determined the "motor points" upon the skin where electrical stimulation would cause different muscles to contract. His book *Physiologie des mouvements* has not been excelled since in his particular field. But it is important to realize just what it was he did. Duchenne verified the inferences about potential muscle actions that had (or could have) been made by simple observation. He used an electrical stimulator as a substitute for a *motor* nerve, making a chosen muscle obey *his* will, not the subject's. Thus his method determined his results in the same sense that a lawyer's "leading question" may determine the answer of a witness.

Nonetheless the Duchennian method of experiment did add very considerably to the sum of kinesiological knowledge. The confirmation by one method of a conclusion reached by another method is an essential step in any kind of physical investigation. Apart from this, Duchenne's electro-stimulation became the basis of valuable procedures in the diagnosis and treatment of many forms of neuromuscular disorder.

ELECTRICAL (2). The second way of using electrical apparatus is as a substitute for a *sensory* nerve, that is, to tell us when a muscle is actually contracting in voluntary, habitual or reflex movements. It is based upon the discovery, nearly 40 years ago, that a contracting muscle fibre is like an active nerve fibre in that it undergoes a recordable change in electrical potential. The development of amplifying and recording electrical apparatus during the second world war made it possible to apply this discovery easily and widely for the study of muscular activity in living human beings. The gathering of information by this means is *electromyography*, now the standard method of experiment in this field.

In electromyography, an electrode is applied either upon the skin (surface electrode) or within selected parts of a muscle (needle or wire electrode). Each of such electrodes is connected to a "channel" of the recording apparatus, the electromyograph. Hence we speak of 1-channel, 2-channel and even 32-channel electromyographs. These multi-channel instruments allow us to study the contraction and relaxation of many muscles during some chosen movement or postural state of a joint. In this way we can find out how muscles are coördinated in action as well as whether or not some particular muscle capable of acting is in fact used. For more information about electromyography the reader is referred to the books listed at the end of this chapter.

Theory

Observation and experiment give us facts. But facts alone are not enough. Indeed, we can have so many facts that they confuse rather than help our understanding of them. Here theory comes in.

Astronomy furnishes a very good example. After the Pole, Kopernik (1473–1543), had proposed that certain astronomical facts could be made more understandable by supposing that the earth went round the sun, instead of its being the other way round, some Western Europeans began to examine the actually observed motions of the planets more closely. Particularly good work in this field was done by a Dane, Tycho Brahe (1546–1601). Then a German, Johann Kepler (1571–1630), applied his knowledge of mathematics and found that Brahe's observations could be simply explained by supposing that the planetary paths were ellipses, not circles as Kopernik had thought. This was a *kinematic* postulate, referring only to the path of a planet, not to why it followed this path and no other. Next came Galileo Galilei (1564–1642), who was an experimentalist. He discovered the principle of the pendulum, and therefore a way of measuring time accurately over short periods. Using this, he found that bodies moving freely under their own weight did so with constant acceleration. At the end of this line came Isaac Newton (1642–1727), who invented the binomial theorem and the differential and integral calculi. Armed with these weapons he looked at Kepler's observational results in the light of Galileo's experimental findings. He showed that the second of these could be used to explain the first if he assumed that every planet tended to move in a straight line by itself but was constrained to move around the sun by a constant acceleration towards it. That is, Newton combined two earlier theories about seemingly different kinds of things by making each of them follow from a more general and purely mathematical theory relating forces and kinds of motion (rectilinear and curvilinear) to each other. He founded modern mechanics.

We have chosen Newton, rather than that other great Englishman, William Harvey (1578–1657), to illustrate the place of theory in combining the results of observation and experiment. Newton's work is obviously particularly relevant to kinesiology. In the study of movements and of the forces that cause them, theory has a double part to play. It enables a mass of anatomical and electromyographical facts to be seen as proceeding from the working of quite simple general laws, and it suggests new lines of investigation that might not be thought of otherwise. For the establishment of this theory mathematics, some of it quite new, is also needed. But the results can be put in simple form, the rigorous proofs required having been already published in specialized journals. In the chapters that follow these results will be used as occasion demands.

The passage from observation through experiment to theory is, then, followed by a passage back to new observation. We have a *methodological cycle* of inquiry in kinesiology as in other branches of knowledge. For example, when we come to consider the movements of the tendons of penniform muscles we shall find that the theory of muscular action in general leads us to have another look at the exact form and arrangement of the individual fibres of these muscles, an investigation that might otherwise be considered trivial.

Kinesiology can be divided into two parts, general and special. General kinesiology deals with the types of movement actually found, with the theory linking many of these types together, with the different ways in which muscles can act and with the theory of both potential and actual muscle action. Special kinesiology deals with the movements and muscles found in particular parts of the body. Both divisions of the subject are related to its application to problems of daily life, industrial and medical. We shall, therefore, consider it under each of these headings, in the order just indicated. This explains the plan of the book.

GENERAL READING

Barnett, C.H., Davies, D.V. and MacConaill, M.A. *Synovial Joints: Their Structure and Mechanics.* London, Longmans Green and Co. Ltd., 1961.

Basmajian, J.V. *Muscles Alive: Their Functions Revealed by Electromyography.* 3rd Ed., Baltimore, Williams & Wilkins Co., 1974.

Basmajian, J.V. *Grant's Method of Anatomy.* 9th Ed., Baltimore, Williams & Wilkins Co., 1975.

Bernstein, N. *The Co-ordination and Regulation of Movements.* 1st English Ed., Oxford, New York, Toronto, Pergamon Press, 1967.

Close, J.R. *Motor Function in the Lower Extremity.* Springfield, Illinois, Charles C. Thomas, 1964.

Duchenne, G.B.A. *Physiologie des mouvements.* 1867. Transl. by E.G. Kaplan, Philadelphia and London, W.B. Saunders, 1949.

Steindler, A. *Kinesiology of the Human Body.* Springfield, Illinois, Charles C Thomas, 1955.

Williams, M. and Lissner, H.R. *Biomechanics of Human Motion.* Philadelphia and London, W.B. Saunders, 1962.

Part Two
GENERAL LAWS OF KINESIOLOGY

TWO

Basic Types of Movement of Bone

Every bone moves at some joint. We should, then, speak of a movement *of* that bone *on* some other *at* that joint, for example a flexion of one phalanx on another at an interphalangeal joint. But long-established custom allows us to speak *of* a joint, and we shall do so when convenient.*

The movements of a bone in space can, however, be studied independently from those it carries out inside the joint *at* which it moves. The movements of a bone can often be studied in the living subject directly; in addition, X-ray studies, both still and cinematographic, increase our knowledge of these movements and give us knowledge of the movements of those other bones that cannot be observed directly.

We can refer to the study of bone movements as *osteokinematics*, the word kinematics meaning the study of movements. (Similarly, movements within joints can be referred to as *arthrokinematics*.)

OSTEOKINEMATICS

We study osteokinematics in order to find the smallest number of types of movement that are sufficient to account for the actual movement of any bone moving at some joint of which it forms a part. Any such actual movement will consist of one or more such basic movements, alone, together or in

---

*The terms used for movements at particular joints will be those adopted by the American Academy of Orthopaedic Surgery, later approved by the British Orthopaedic Association.

13

succession. The actual movement of the bone in space will, of course, depend upon the association of its "private" movements with those of bones moving at other joints. We shall, therefore, consider only the basic types of movement in this chapter.

Spin and Swing

There are only two basic ways in which a bone can move, namely, by spinning or by swinging. They are both types of what the engineer calls "rotation" around some axis. However, medical custom has confined the use of "rotation" to what is called medio-lateral (internal-external) rotation, so that the terms spin and swing are necessary. They are also well-known English words.* To define them we must first define what is meant by a mechanical axis.

In osteokinematics we can always imagine any bone to be replaced by a rod, this rod moving at the joint at which the bone moves. In the special cases of the humerus and femur we replace the *shafts* of these bones by rods that pass through the heads of these bones, as shown in fig. 2.1; the reason for this will be given in the next chapter. Thus we reduce osteokinematics to the study of the possible motions of a rod. The *mechanical axis* of a bone is the line running in the middle of the rod from end to end. The rod has some thickness and so has a surface. We can, therefore, take any point on this surface and study its motion also, if need be. We are now ready to define spin and swing.

SPIN. When the *only* motion of our chosen point on the surface is a *rotation around the mechanical axis*, then the rod (with the corresponding bone) undergoes *pure spin*.

SWING. Any movement other than pure spin is a *swing*.

We have thus defined swings by means of spins. We can divide swings into two types, pure and impure.

PURE SWING. If a bone swings without any accompanying spin, the swing is pure.

---

* See Appendix A.

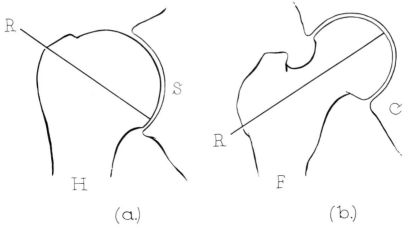

Fig. 2.1. To show the position of a rod (R) replacing one along the shaft of the moving bone at the shoulder and hip joints in kinematical studies. (a) Shoulder: S, scapula; H, humerus. (b) Hip: C, hip bone (os coxae); F, femur.

IMPURE SWING. If a bone swings and also undergoes some spin, the swing is impure.

The movements called internal and external rotation are spins. Ideally, they are pure spins; this is not true in practice, but they approximate well enough to pure spins to serve as examples. A spin must be either clockwise or anticlockwise. Thus medial rotation of the right humerus is anticlockwise if viewed by the possessor of the humerus, and lateral rotation is clockwise from the same point of view. But these two movements will be clockwise and anticlockwise, respectively, if seen by some observer who is looking directly at the lower end of the humerus.

Any point of a bone moving at a joint moves in a curved line, even though the curvature of the line be slight. This is obvious in the case of the larger bones, and is a matter of fundamental importance. Hence all swings are along curved lines, which is indeed the reason for their name. When studying swings, we consider a point on the mechanical axis, *e.g.*, at its extremity. In a pure swing this point moves from its initial to its final position in space along the shortest possible curved line. This line corresponds to a meridian of longitude on a sphere, and to a straight line on a flat surface. In an impure swing the movement is always along some curved line other than the shortest. This corresponds to an *arc* between two points on a flat surface, the line of pure swing corresponding to the *chord* between the same points. For this reason an impure swing is called an *arcuate swing*. A pure swing is called a *cardinal swing* because it is like the movement allowed by a carpenter's ideal hinge (Latin *cardo* = hinge).

Degrees of Freedom

If a bone can swing in one way only or can spin only, it is said to have 1 *degree of freedom* (DF). If it can both spin and swing in one way only *or* if it can swing in two completely distinct ways (see below) but not spin, then it has 2 DF. If it can spin and also swing in two distinct ways, then it has 3 DF. A phalanx of thumb or finger has 1 DF; the radius and the first metacarpal bone have 2 DF; the humerus and the femur have 3 DF.

Two terms require explanation: "way of swing" and "completely distinct ways of swing"; they are best explained by means of an example. If one bone can be flexed upon another then, having been flexed, it can be extended upon the other again. The flexion takes place in one direction, the extension in the reverse direction: the two directions constitute the *way of swing*; in this instance the way of swing is flexion-extension. So also abduction-adduction and mediolateral rotation are ways of swing. If one direction of swing is considered to be positive then the other constituent of the corresponding way of swing is negative. Thus, if flexion be taken as positive then extension is "negative flexion". For example, 20° of flexion (F) followed by 20° of extension ($-$F) is clearly equivalent to 0° of swing, that is (20° F $-$ 20° F).

Two conditions must be fulfilled for two ways of swing to

be completely distinct from each other: (1) the swings must be *cardinal,* and (2) the axis of one way of swing must be at right angles to that of the other way of swing. These conditions are the explicit way of stating something that has been recognised implicitly for centuries. If a bone has only 2 DF then it can carry out cardinal swings around only two axes, and these also are at right angles to each other; this is a conclusion based upon observation and experiments so that fulfilment of the first condition in this case means that the second condition is fulfilled also. The need for stating the second condition arises when a bone has 3 DF. We take the humerus as an example.

We can swing a humerus in two ways: upwards-downwards in flexion-extension and also in abduction-adduction, the axes of motion for these two ways being manifestly at right angles to each other. But we can also swing it upwards-downwards about axes that are intermediate between those of flexion-extension and of abduction-adduction. Why do we not reckon these other ways as so many more degrees of freedom of swing? The answer is because each of these others can be completely defined by means of the first pair (fig. 2.2). As the figure shows, all axes of humeral upwards-downwards swing lie in the same horizontal plane and intersect in a common point. If s-s' be one axis of swing, and if f-f' and a-a' be the flexion-extension and abduction-adduction axes, respectively, then s-s' makes an angle F with f-f' and an angle A with a-a'. These two angles define the axis s-s' completely.

We can go further. When (A + F) = 90° the axis runs in a certain direction; when (A − F) = 90° the axis runs in a direction at right angles to the former (see fig. 2.2). Thus both angles, and therefore both the axes, a-a' and f-f', are necessary and also sufficient for defining the actual axis of cardinal swings, s-s'. When F = 0 the way of swing is flexion-extension and when A = 0 the way of swing is abduction-adduction. When (F + A) = 90° an upward swing will be forwards and outwards; when (F − A) = 90° an upward swing will be forwards and inwards.

There is another type of swing which seems at first to make an addition to the 3 DF at the shoulder and the hip. Take a man who is standing upright with his arm hanging by his side. He can lift the arm upwards and then swing it in a *horizontal* plane, backwards or forwards. This horizontal swing is shown in fig. 2.3. With one exception, such a horizontal swing is *arcuate*, not cardinal, the exception being when the arm is raised until it is horizontal (*i.e.*, parallel with the ground) and kept so throughout the swing (see Chapter 4). In this exceptional case a forward swing is called *horizontal flexion*, and a backward swing is called *horizontal extension*. Does horizontal flexion-extension constitute a 4th DF?

It does not, because a horizontal swing must take place around a *vertical* axis. Now medio-lateral spin of the humeral shaft takes place around a vertical axis when the arm is hanging by the side. Hence a horizontal swing does not add to

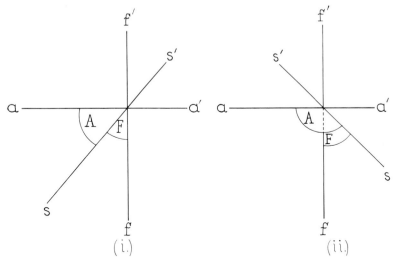

Fig. 2.2. To show how an actual axis *(s-s')* of humeral vertical swing can be defined by means of two fixed axes at right angles to each other: *a-a'*, medio-lateral axis; *f-f'*, antero-posterior axis. Explanation of angles A and F in text. (i) A + F = 90°; (ii) A + F greater than 90°.

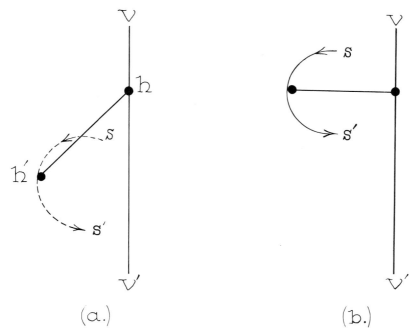

(a.)   (b.)

Fig. 2.3. To illustrate horizontal swing. VV′, vertical axis around which swing occurs; hh′, rod representing humerus; ss′, path of swing. In (a) the humerus has been abducted through less than a right angle; in (b) it has been abducted through a right angle. In both cases the path of swing is in a horizontal plane.

the number of axes that define the 3 DF of movements of the humerus. The importance of this fact will be stressed in Chapter 4, as it applies to all joints having 3 DF.

The Ovoid of Movement

Much space has been given to the subject of axes of swing because the movements of bones are often described in terms of them and it is also often convenient to do so. But if we wish to understand many important facts of osteokinematics we must express them in terms of what has been, and still is, often called the "sphere of movement" of a bone and is

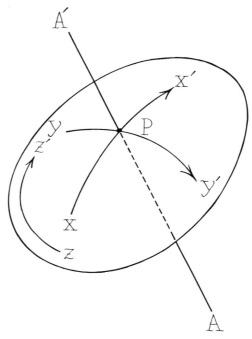

Fig. 2.4. An ovoid of motion. P is a point on the mechanical axis (AA′) of a bone moving in space. XX′, YY′ and ZZ′, three possible paths of P on the ovoid of motion outlined.

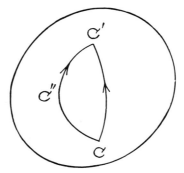

Fig. 2.5. A chordal and an arcuate path between the same two points on an ovoid of motion. CC′ is the chordal; CC″C′ is the arcuate path. The arcuate is longer than the chordal, which is the shortest path between the first and last points.

pure swing – chord
impure swing – arcuate

better called the *ovoid of movement*. To use this concept is
in fact simpler than to use axes of swing for describing bone
movements, for only the *mechanical axis* of the bone itself is
required, together with one point on the surface of the bone.

If we take some point on the mechanical axis and follow its
movements of swing we find that each of these is a curved line
in space. The complete set of lines of swing lies on a virtual
("imaginary") surface (fig. 2.4). This surface is always convex
on that side which is further from the joint. It may be large
or small, depending on the amount of swing allowed to the
bone in different directions. It is not like a piece of the surface
of a sphere; it is more like a piece of eggshell, the curvature
of which varies from point to point in a way difficult to express
exactly in simple mathematical terms; hence we refer to this
surface as the *ovoid of movement*.

In fig. 2.4, P is a point on the mechanical axis AA'. The

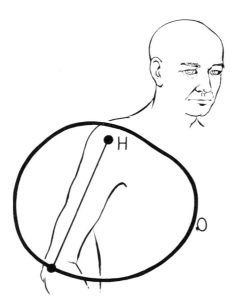

Fig. 2.6. An outline of the ovoid of motion (O) of the humerus (H) at the
shoulder (after Benninghoff-Goerttler, *Lehrb. d. Anatomie des Menschen*,
9th ed., Bd. 1, 1964).

figure shows some of the possible paths on the ovoid of movement that P moves along during a cardinal swing (if AA′ has 2 or 3 DF of movement). In fig. 2.5 two paths are shown; one, CC′, is a *chordal path*, corresponding to a cardinal swing of AA′; the other, CC″C′, is an arcuate path between the first and last points of the chordal.

The shape of the boundary of the ovoid will, of course, differ from bone to bone. That of the humeral ovoid is shown in fig. 2.6. It is to be noted that this boundary is that of the ovoid of movement of the humerus moving on the scapula at the shoulder (glenohumeral) joint.

The concept of the ovoid of movement is a most important one. It enables us to describe the motions of a bone entirely in terms of a point on the mechanical axis of that bone moving on the ovoid.

The full theory of kinesiology derived from ovoids of motion will be found in Appendix A. Its algebra may seem strange at first, but it is really quite simple. Its more important consequences will be stated after two basic terms in it have been defined.

Conjunct and Adjunct Rotations

There are two basic types of rotation (spin), conjunct and adjunct. Each may be either *clockwise* or *anticlockwise*, as seen by some observer. For brevity, these will be denoted by CWR and ACWR, respectively.

The *sense* of either a rotation or an arcuate swing is either CWR or ACWR.

Conjunct Rotation. If the passage of a bone along a single path or a set of successive paths *necessarily* involves a CWR or an ACWR of that bone, then the rotation is called a *conjunct rotation*, because it is conjoined with the arcuate swing.

Adjunct Rotation. Any other rotation of a bone is called an *adjunct rotation*, because it is adjoined *either* to no rotation at all (producing a pure spin) or to a conjunct rotation.

Antispin. Any adjunct rotation added to a conjunct rotation of opposite sense will be called an *antispin*. Thus, an adjunct CWR added to a conjunct ACWR is an antispin.

Clearly, the amount of an antispin will determine whether it diminishes, nullifies, or even reverses a conjunct rotation — more strictly, the effect of the conjunct rotation on the bone.

Swings and Conjunct Rotations

There is only one chordal path for any point in a moving bone between its initial and its final position; and a bone moving along a chordal path suffers no conjunct rotation. In these two respects a chordal path is the equivalent of a linear path on a flat surface. As we have seen, such a movement is called a chordal or "cardinal" swing, that is, a pure swing. It is a fact of biomechanics that cardinal swings occur only at joints of at least two degrees of freedom.

An arcuate swing is always accompanied by a conjunct rotation, although the *effect* of this rotation may be increased, diminished, nullified or reversed by an antispin. The *sense* and amount of the conjunct rotation are always determined by the initial and final angles that the arc of motion makes with its chord *and by them alone*. These angles may both lie on the same side of the chord; or they may lie on different sides of the chord. This, in turn, depends upon whether the arc belongs to one or other of two fundamental types, the unisensual or the bisensual (fig. 2.7).

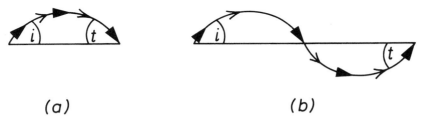

(a)   **(b)**

Fig. 2.7. Conjunct rotation caused by (a) unisensual and (b) bisensual arcuate swing. *i*: initial, and *t*: terminal angle between arc of swing and its chord (shown by straight line). Compare positions of apex of the moving triangle.

A *unisensual* swing (or arc) is one whose initial and terminal angles are both on the *same* side of the chord. Hence, if it begins as either clockwise or anticlockwise it will end in the same sense. If i and t be its initial and terminal angles, respectively, then the total conjunct rotation is $(i+t)$; and it will be either a CWR or an ACWR.

A *bisensual* swing (or arc) is one whose initial and terminal angles are on *opposite* sides of the chord. Hence:

(i) the arc must cross the chord *at least* once; and

(ii) the terminal part of the swing (arc) must be of *opposite sense* to its initial part (otherwise it would not cross the chord); this is why it has been called bisensual.

If again i and t denote the initial and terminal angles, respectively, then the total conjunct rotation will be $(i-t)$, not $(i+t)$. This is because the "oppositeness" of the sense of one part of an arc to another is denoted by the minus (negative) sign; thus, we could write *qualitatively* ACWR = -CWR.

It follows that the sense of the conjunct rotation caused by a bisensual swing may be that of a CWR, an ACWR, or neither (i.e., 0°). Suppose, for example, that i is 30° and that the arc is initially one of CWR. Then for t-values of 15°, 30° and 45° the conjunct rotations will be, respectively, 15°, 0° and -15°; the last being an ACWR. The cases in which the rotation is 0 will be considered below (p. 26).

The Effects of Adjunct Rotations

Adjunct rotations applied to an arcuately swinging bone are either cospins or antispins. A *cospin* has the *same* sense (CWR or ACWR) as the swing; an *antispin* has the *opposite* sense. If a denotes a cospin of a certain amount, then $-a$ denotes an antispin of the same amount (fig. 2.8).

If the total amount of the conjunct rotation by itself would be c then the total rotation r produced by an adjunct swing is $(c+a)$ for a cospin and $(c-a)$ for an antispin. There is a limit to the value of r: in no case can the *total* rotation exceed that permitted by the joint without an adjunct rotation. This limita-

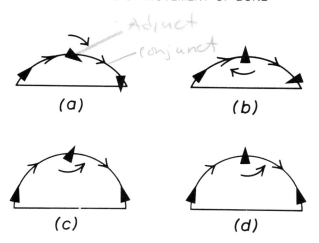

Fig. 2.8. Effect of type of adjunct rotation on conjunct rotation. (a) Augmenting type (cospin). (b) Reversing. (c) Gradual nullifying, and (d) Immediate nullifying types (antispins). The *small curved arrows* show the sense of adjunct rotation.

tion is *biomechanical*, being due to the capsule and other ligaments of the joint at which the motion takes place.

Take as an example the cases in which $c = 30°$ and the adjunct rotation has values of $15°$ (cospin) or $-30°$ or $-45°$. Then the corresponding values of r will be, respectively, $45°$ (augmentation), $0°$ (nullification) and $-15°$ (reversal). An adjunct rotation of $-10°$ would make $r = 20°$ (diminution).

Nullifying antispins are of special importance. They are of two kinds: *gradual* and *immediate*. The gradual type achieves its total effect only at the end of the swing. The immediate type both produces its effect at the start of the swing and is operative as a nullifier throughout the whole swing. In this way it prevents any rotation of the bone at any stage of the swing. An example of an immediate antispin is shown in figure 2.8, and an important movement involving one will be described in the next section but one.*

---

*In mathematical terms the distinction between gradual and immediate nullifying antispins is this. For both types $\int da = - \int dc$; but for the immediate type we have also $da/dx = -dc/dx$, where x is the total length of the arc of swing.

Quasichordal Swings

Any swing for which the total rotation is 0 is called a *quasi-chordal* swing, because the result of the swing is *as if* the bone had moved from its initial to its final position along a chord — *quasi* = as if. Such a swing may be bisensual, or a suitable antispin may take place during it. An example of a bisensual quasichordal swing that the reader can easily study will now be given, the experiments being made on a finger.

As a preliminary, we first note that IP and MP are widely used contractions for "interphalangeal" and "metacarpophalangeal", respectively. We also note that the fingers from index through anulus have each a pair of interosseus muscles acting on them. These can be called the *radial* and the *ulnar* interosseus muscles, denoted by RI and UI, respectively. (These names avoid the confusion caused by the different numbering of the palmar interossei on the two sides of the North Atlantic.)

First extend both IP joints and the MP joint of, say, an index finger; but keep the IP joints fully extended during all that follows. There are two ways of fully flexing the finger at the MP joint. One is by a cardinal swing; this is what textbooks call flexion-motion. The other way is to begin the flexion by swinging the finger through an arc which is convex either toward the ulnar or towards the radial side. Do this for the index and continue to move it until it is fully flexed. You will see that the initial arc cannot be continued beyond about semiflexion (with either an ulnar or a radial deviation, depending on the arc). After that point the finger travels in an arc of *opposite sense to the first;* and ends its course in full flexion.

During the second mode of flexion the conjunct rotations of the finger can be easily observed. That of the first stage is reversed during the second stage. In short, any of the fingers can be brought to full flexion either by a cardinal swing or by one of two bisensual swings, each of the latter being, therefore, quasichordal.

The part played by the musculature is easy to understand. It is well established that if the IP joints are kept extended then the MP joint is fully flexed by the combined action of the RI and the UI. Each of these muscles acting alone causes an arcuate swing that is convex towards its own side, but, as the experiment shows, there is a limit to the arc. After this limit has been reached the other muscle of the pair comes into action and reverses the direction of the arcuate motion; and, of course the sense of the finger's conjunct rotation. In the case of the 5th finger (digit V or *digitus minimus*) the abductor-flexion mass takes the place of an ulnar interosseus muscle.

Revolutions

So far we have been talking (or thinking) about *open* swings, i.e., those that do not end where they began. To complete our study of basic motions of bones, we must consider *closed* swings, those that do end where they began. They are of constant occurrence in work and in play, hence their importance.

We emphasize that closed swings are basic motions. They occur along arcs whose associated conjunct rotation is (theoretically!) 360°, though such a rotation is not in fact permitted. No closed swing is a chordal one, though both classes of them are quasichordal. They can be described as successions of other basic motions; but this is a needless complication.

Revolution is the name for a closed swing. It is used in the sense in which we say that the earth spins around its own axis. The orbit of any point of a revolving bone lies in a plane which cuts that plane's ovoid of motion along the line of that orbit; and the nearer the point is to the joint at which the revolution occurs the smaller is its orbit. These two facts are often expressed by saying that the bone describes a cone in space, but this concept is unnecessary for understanding revolutions. For all purposes except a mathematical analysis it is enough to know (and verify experimentally on yourself and others!) the following facts:

i) The orbits of the extra-articular extremity of a revolving bone are either a *circle* of maximal radius or lie within that circle. These "inner" orbits may be circular, or oval, or of some other shape.

ii) Revolutions can take place only at joints having at least two degrees of freedom.

iii) If any bone revolves, then any bone more distal from the "joint of revolution" than it will revolve also in an orbit *of similar shape;* the importance of this fact will be pointed out later.

iv) The plane of a revolution is *normal* ("at right angles everywhere") to the axis around which the maximal circle of revolution takes place, this axis passing through the center of that circle. Such planes are best named as vertical, horizontal or oblique with respect to the space outside the body; and can be specified further as anterior, lateral, posterior, etc. with respect to the body.

v) The range of planes is greater for joints of 3 degrees of freedom than for those of 2 degrees; and the shoulder joint (i.e., the humerus) has the greatest range of all — as the reader probably knows.

Visible revolutions are all that need concern us; they will be named after the parts that revolve, the joints involved being given in parentheses. In the upper limb there are the thumb (1st carpometacarpal) the fingers (MP joints), the hand as a whole (radiocarpal) and the whole limb (shoulder). In the lower limb there are the limb itself (hip) and the foot (ankle); the latter is difficult and needs practice to carry out smoothly, and is more easily seen in its reversed form (leg moving on foot). Finally, there are the trunk (thoracolumbar vertebral series) and the head (cervical series). At all these joints, revolution can be clockwise or anticlockwise.

There are *two kinds of revolution,* perigyration and circumduction. Circular revolutions are enough to show their difference.*

Perigyration (fig. 2.9 a) is a revolution during which there is no rotation of the bone from start to finish. During it an imme-

---

*In existing textbooks "revolution" is called circumduction and is not analyzed further. Here "circumduction" is applied to the motion that can occur at *all* joints at which rotation is possible. Sathe (1955) calls it "circumrotation"; this offends against the meaning of rotation (spin) accepted by kinesiologists everywhere.

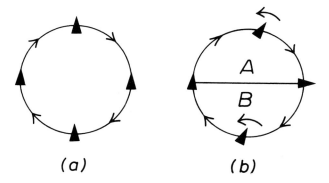

Fig. 2.9. The two types of Revolution. (a) Perigyration: no conjunct rotation. (b) Circumduction: diminished conjunct rotation in first phase (A), undoing of the rotation in second stage (B); *small arrows* show constant sense of the antispin.

diate nullifying antispin acts continuously on the humerus or femur, for it occurs only at a shoulder or hip joint. We have *modified perigyration* of the limb if the antecubitum (forearm and hand) is allowed pronation or supination during the humeral motion; but demonstration of the humeral pure perigyration is, of course, most easy when the antecubitum is, say, kept semipronated.

There is always some motion at the acromioclavicular and sternoclavicular joints during both perigyration and humeral circumduction; this increases as the plane of these motions moves upwards.

Circumduction (fig. 2.9 b) differs from perigyration by having two phases, the *first* and the *return* phases; each phase extends over one-half of the closed swing. In the first phase a gradual diminishing antispin acts on the bone to modify the total conjunct rotation that would otherwise occur (i.e., 180°). In the second phase this antispin continues and the bone's rotation is completely undone.

The maximal conjunct rotation caused by the first phase occurs in the circle of revolution of greatest diameter; and diminishes as the diameter diminishes. It also diminishes at the shoulder and hip joints according to the extent to which the humerus and femur have been first rotated in the same sense as that of the circumduction to be carried out.

The maximal rotation of the humerus is about 90°; of the femur somewhat under 90°; of the thumb and fingers 45°; and of the whole hand, not more than 30°. It is much easier to perigyrate the humerus than to circumduct it. This can be ascribed reasonably to the biomechanical fact that the purpose of a humeral circumduction can be achieved by a combination of humeral perigyration with pronation-supination of the forearm and/or circumduction of the whole hand at the radiocarpal joint.

The Neutral Positions of Bones and Joints

The Neutral Position of a bone or joint is the position from which its movements are named and should be measured, or tested in some other way. The various neutral positions can be seen directly by looking at a vertically standing person whose head, neck, trunk and limbs satisfy the following conditions —

1) The thighs and legs are vertical;

2) The feet point directly forward;

3) The eyes look directly forward;

4) The neck and trunk are vertical and untwisted;

5) All the parts of the upper limb are *pendent*, that is, hanging vertically downward and in line with one another;

6) The forearm (and hand) are *semipronated*, so that the palm faces the thigh;

7) The *thumb* is in contact with the radial side of the palm (an exception to 5, strictly speaking).

The neutral position is that of *full extension* of the parts below the elbow; of nearly full extension of the hip and knee; and of the head and vertebral column when loads are carried on the head.

The neutral position is also called the *zero position* when measurements are taken from it.

REFERENCES

Sathe, Y.S. (1955) Circumrotation. *J. Anat. Med. Soc. India*, June, 14-17.

THREE

Basic Types of Movements at Joints

We shall consider first and foremost the basic movements at *synovial* joints. This is the most frequent type of joint and, in any case, there is always a synovial joint involved in the movement of any bone. It is presumed that the reader already has some knowledge of the structure of synovial joints, so that all that need be done here is to point out what parts of this structure are important in the present connection.

The Shapes of Articular Surfaces

No articular surface is flat; neither is any surface like a flat surface that has been rolled up to form part of the surface of a cylinder or cone. What are called "plane" surfaces in the standard textbooks are always slightly curved in one of the two ways now to be described.

(1) OVOID SURFACES. These are either *convex* in all directions or *concave* in all directions, that is, they are like either the outer or the inner surface of a piece of eggshell. From the kinematical point of view they are equivalent and are both called "surfaces of *positive* curvature", or "synclastic" surfaces. The outer and inner surfaces of a sphere are classical examples of this type. But every part of the surface of a sphere has the same curvature at every point, whereas articular surfaces have not. In this respect convex and concave articular surfaces are like a piece of eggshell, not a sphere,

31

for the piece of shell also has a curvature that varies from point to point. This is why such articular surfaces are called ovoid (fig. 3.1). The imaginary surface on which any point on the mechanical axis of a bone moves is of this type; hence the name "ovoid of movement". Even the surfaces found in the so-called ball-and-socket joints are of this type, not of a spherical type. This is why such joints are called "spheroidal" —"rather but not quite like spherical joints".

(2) SELLAR SURFACES. The other major type of articular surface is the *sellar*, from the Latin word for saddle (*sella*). A section of this kind of surface in one direction is of convex outline; a section cut at right angles to the first direction is of concave outline (fig. 3.2). The metacarpal surface of the trapezium is a classical example of a saddle surface. Other examples are the hamate surface of the triquetrum, the cuboid surface of the calcaneus and the fibular surface of the talus. It is indeed a very common type of surface, and its significance will be stated in the next chapter. This type of surface is one of "negative" curvature.

There is another way of classifying surfaces, namely, as *male* and *female*, a custom first introduced by engineers. A convex surface is male, a concave one is female. What, then,

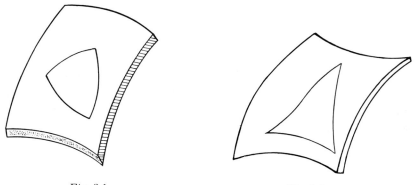

Fig. 3.1.   Fig. 3.2.

Fig. 3.1. Part of an ovoid surface with a chordal triangle drawn on it.
Fig. 3.2. Part of a sellar surface with a chordal triangle drawn on it.

about saddle surfaces? Which of two saddle surfaces forming part of a joint is to be called male, which female? The question is answered by taking another look at ovoid surfaces forming part of a single articulation. One of these is male (convex), the other female (concave), and *the female surface is always of smaller area than the male.* Hence the larger of our two sellar surfaces is called male and the smaller is called female.

The Congruence of Articular Surfaces

Every (synovial) joint contains at least one *mating pair* of articular surfaces, one of these being male, the other female. When there is only one mating pair the joint is called *simple*. When there is more than one mating pair the joint is called *compound*. When there is an intra-articular disc the joint is called *complex*.

When one bone articulates with two others within one and the same compound joint it will have *two* articular surfaces, one for each of the other two bones. We thus have *two mating pairs*. For example, the lower end of the radius articulates with the scaphoid and the lunate bones of the radio-carpal joint. Each of these two bones has a male ovoid surface which moves on a corresponding *and separate* female ovoid surface on the lower end of the radius. Thus we have the two mating pairs that constitute the radioscaphoid and the radio-lunate joints. There is an important rule governing the behaviour of adjacent mating pairs within any compound joint: *No male surface of one mating pair comes into articulation with the female surface of another mating pair,* and conversely. The mating pairs are, so to speak, married till death do them part! Accordingly, many basic features of intra-articular movement can be studied on single mating pairs of the appropriate form, ovoid or sellar.

In all positions of a mating pair except one, the mating pairs fit each other badly—they are not fully *congruent*. The position in which they are fully congruent is called the *close-packed position*. In this special position the female articular surface fits the corresponding (apposed) part of the male surface point-for-point. Moreover, the chief ligaments of the joint are so arranged that they screw the male and female surfaces together in the close-packed position in such a way that they cannot be pulled apart—whence the name. All other positions of a joint are called *loose-packed*. In the close-packed position we no longer have two bones functionally, only one, because they have been temporarily screwed together. It follows that the number of degrees of freedom vanishes to 0, so far as concerns movement of one of these bones upon the other. The degrees of freedom (1, 2, or 3) will not be exhibited until the joint is brought into loose-pack or, of course, until the joint is moved out of close-pack. The difference between close-pack and loose-pack is shown in fig. 3.3.

Movements of Female Ovoid Surfaces

In this section a female ovoid surface will be called simply a "female surface".

A female surface can both *spin* and *slide* on its male mate; sliding is illustrated in fig. 3.4. Both these types of

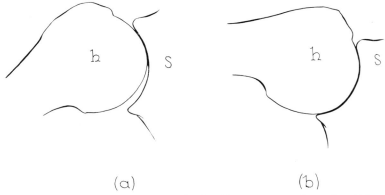

(a)　　　　　　　　　　　　　(b)

Fig. 3.3. Diagram of glenohumeral (shoulder) joint to show the difference between loose-pack position (a) and close-pack position (b). h, humerus; s, scapula. Observe that the humerus descends on the glenoid cavity as it comes into close-pack.

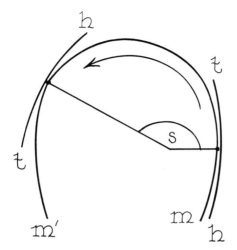

Fig. 3.4.

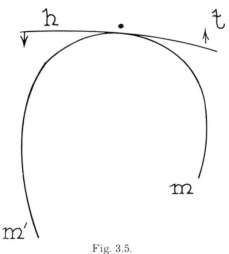

Fig. 3.5.

Fig. 3.4. To show angle of rotation (s) due to slide of a female surface (th) upon a male surface (mm′). Arrow shows direction of slide.

Fig. 3.5. To illustrate rocking (rolling) of the female surface of fig. 3.4 upon the male surface.

movement are combined in a hinge joint, separable in joints of 2 and 3 DF. In addition, a female surface can *rock* to a small but sensible extent on the male, except when the joint is close-packed and there is no room for rocking! This last movement is illustrated in fig. 3.5.

Except at the very beginning and the very end of a movement, rocking is always accompanied by sliding. A female surface always rocks in the direction in which the sliding is taking place. Thus if it be sliding forward then it rocks forward also; that is, its "leading" edge approaches the male surface and its "trailing" edge is lifted further from that surface. Hence *during a sliding movement the female surface constantly approaches the male in the direction of motion.* This clearly is a result of the incongruity of the male and female surfaces in loose-pack. It is associated with the lubrication of the joint by synovial fluid.

The mechanical axis of the "female" bone is swung through space as a result of the combination of rocking and sliding of the female surface on the male, and its total angular displacement can be analyzed as an addition of the results of these two components (fig. 3.6). As the figure shows, the effect of rocking is to supplement that of sliding. If a be the total angular displacement of the mechanical axis, s the displacement due to sliding and r that due to rocking, we have:

$$a = r + s$$

This fact makes for economy in the amount of cartilage used

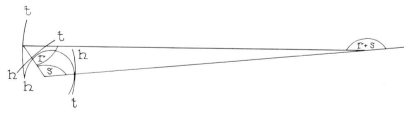

Fig. 3.6. To illustrate the combined effect (r + s) of the angle of rotation due to slide (s) and that due to rocking (r) of the female surface upon the male surface of fig. 3.4.

for making articular surfaces, as will be illustrated in connection with male ovoid surfaces.

Movements of Male Ovoid Surfaces

In this section we shall use "male surface" for male ovoid surface.

Like female surfaces, male surfaces can both slide and spin. In addition, they can *roll* upon the female surface. Rolling is always accompanied by sliding, except at the very beginning and end of a movement, and, of course, rolling does not take place when the joint is in close-pack.

Rolling is the principal movement of a male surface, other than spinning. The direction of the slide that accompanies the roll is *opposite* to that of the roll. For example, when a lateral femoral condyle rolls forwards (as in extension) it also slides backwards.

The mechanical axis of a "male" bone is swung through space mainly by the rolling movement of the male surface. The effect of the sliding movement supplements that of the roll in this case (fig. 3.7), just as the rocking movement supplements the effect of the slide in the "female" case. We have, therefore, the same kind of equation in the male case as in the female:

$$a = r + s$$

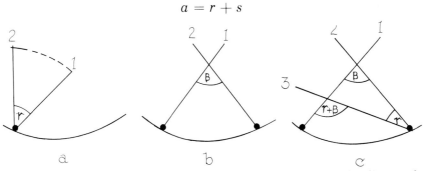

Fig. 3.7. The effect of rolling (a), sliding (b) and combined rolling and sliding (c) upon the axis of a male bone moving upon a female surface. The letters indicate angles; the numbers indicate successive positions of the long axis of the bone.

In the male case r stands for the angular displacement (swing) due to the roll-component of a non-spin movement. There is no reason why we should not also talk of a "female roll" instead of a "rock", so that the r in our equation stands for the same thing—as it does in practice. The *relative* displacement of the "male" and "female" mechanical axes is the same whether it be brought about by movement of one bone, of the other or of both.

The effect of the roll-slide combination in making for economical use of articular cartilage is well seen at the glenohumeral (shoulder) joint. For example, in abduction of the humerus the humeral head not only rolls upwards but also slides downwards upon the curved glenoid surface of the scapula. The total swing is some 90°. Were it not for the slide, the articular cartilage of the humeral head would be required to cover about 25% of a sphere, *i.e.*, one-quarter of 360°. As it is, 20% coverage is enough. This should be contrasted with the hip joint, in which the female surface is so shaped that the sliding of the femoral head in abduction is more restricted than that of the humeral head in the similar movement. Consequently, femoral abduction at the hip joint is much more restricted than humeral at the shoulder joint, about 48° as compared with 90°, respectively.

Flexion-Extension of Femur and Humerus

The femur and humerus are noteworthy in that they perform the movements called pure flexion and pure extension by means of *spins* within the hip and shoulder joints, respectively, not by rolling and sliding. This is because the *true mechanical axis* of each of these bones is mostly intra-articular and makes a marked angle with the mechanical axis of the corresponding shaft (figs. 3.8 and 3.9). This is a matter of importance when we have to consider the rôles of individual muscles in connection with the aforesaid joints. At the moment we are concerned with movements alone.

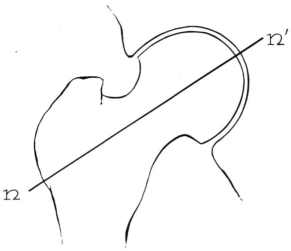

Fig. 3.8. Diagram of the upper end of the femur (femorellum) to show that the long axis of the neck (nn') is the true mechanical axis for the femur at the hip and that the movements called flexion and extension are really spins, not swings.

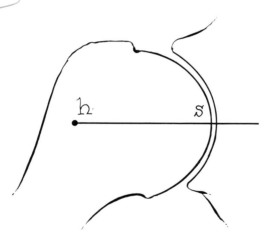

Fig. 3.9. Diagram of glenohumeral joint to show that its true mechanical axis (hs) is normal (perpendicular) to the areas of contact of the male (humeral) and female (glenoid) surfaces, not an axis through the shaft of the humerus; hs is the axis of the humerellum.

The case of the femur is the more obvious. From our present point of view this bone consists primarily of the head, neck and greater trochanter, these constituting the system that performs the movements at the hip joint. The shaft of the bone is merely a lever upon which certain muscles act to move the primary part, which we can call the *femorellum*. The neck of the femur is, then, the "shaft" of the femorellum. This "shaft" is more or less permanently abducted from the midline of the trunk. What we call "abduction" and "adduction" at the hip are really increases or decreases of the amount of this abduction. The movements called medial and lateral "rotation of the femur" are really nearly horizontal forward and backward swings, respectively, of the femorellum. Using the tip of the greater trochanter as a reference point, we can then say that the so-called flexion and extension of the femur are backward and forward *spins*, respectively, of the femorellum upon the acetabular (female) articular surfaces.

In the humerus the head and the greater tuberosity correspond to the femoral head and greater trochanter. The system composed of these parts is what actually moves upon the glenoid cavity; we can call it the *humerellus*. The humerellus, when at rest, will have a mechanical axis that will be normal (perpendicular) to the glenoid surface at the point (small area) of contact of the two bones, as shown in fig. 15. It is upon this axis that the muscles immediately around the shoulder joint, *e.g.*, the supraspinatus, really work. During abduction at the shoulder the humerellus slides downwards upon the glenoid cavity, so that the mechanical axis will change its position as shown in fig. 3.10. This is of importance in connection with the action of the stabilizing muscles of the joint, as will be shown in Chapter 8. The change in position of the axis is a result of a combined sliding and rolling of the humeral head upon the scapula. Taking the uppermost facet of the greater tuberosity as a reference point, we can say that the so-called flexion and extension of the humerus are

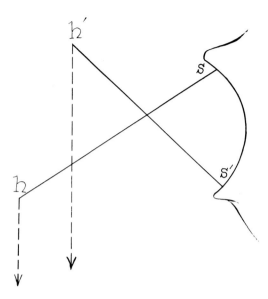

Fig. 3.10. To show the change in position of the mechanical axis of the humerellum at the shoulder joint as it passes from the pendent position (hs) to that of abduction (h's'). Compare with fig. 3.9. The arrows show the direction of the pull of gravity.

backward and forward *spins* of the humerellus upon the glenoid surface of the scapula. The humerellar mechanical axis is, then, like the femorellar axis in that both are, so to speak, already considerably "pre-abducted" from the midline of the trunk—strictly, from its midplane. This fact tends to be masked, in the case of the humerellus, by the relatively great length of the humeral shaft when the arm is pendent, *i.e.*, hanging by the side of the body.

Condylar Joints

One bone may articulate with another either by a single surface or by two *distinct* articular surfaces—never by more than two. When we have an articulation by two distinct surfaces it is called a "condylar joint" or, better, a *bicondylar joint*. Each mating surface is called a "condyle", whether it be male or female. This type of joint is very common, the knee being only one example. The articulation between skull and lower jaw is of this kind, as are the synovial articulations between all the vertebrae except the atlanto-axial. Even though descriptive anatomy talks, for example, of two temporomandibular joints there is only one joint functionally, for the left mandibular head cannot move without the right head's moving also. The upper and lower radio-ulnar joints constitute a single bicondylar articulation for pronation-supination. So also the subtalar and sustentaculotalar joints constitute a bicondylar joint between talus and calcaneus for the purpose of inversion and eversion of the "free" foot. This bicondylar joint is remarkably like that between the radius and the ulna, the head of talus corresponding to that of radius, and calcaneus corresponding to ulna in those cases when ulna moves on radius in pronation-supination.

Bicondylar joints always have 2 DF; in this respect they differ from hinge joints with which they might at first be functionally confused. *Pure spin is never found at these joints* although rotation of one or the other of the mating bones can take place around an axis between the condyles.

There is a variant of the bicondylar type of joint in which one bone mates by distinct articular facets with two other bones that are side by side. We may call this kind of joint *paracondylar*. One example is the humero-radio-ulnar part of the elbow joint, in which the humerus articulates with two other bones. Another is the radiocarpal joint in which the radius articulates with both the scaphoid and the lunate bones. In each case the paracondylar arrangement permits a movement that would otherwise be impossible. At the elbow the radial head can be spun on the humeral capitulum without involvement of the ulna. At the wrist the scaphoid and lunate, notably the former, can be spun on the radius in such a way that the transverse carpal arch is deepened during palmar (volar) flexion and flattened during dorsiflexion—as is verified by X-ray cinematography. This deepening and flattening of the arch is assisted by rotations of the triquetrum in opposite senses to those of the scaphoid, but the scaphoid plays the more important part.

A Note on Nomenclature

In this chapter we have used the engineer's term "mating pairs" for the combination of a male and a female articular surface. Henceforward we shall use the term *conarticular surfaces* instead (MacConaill, 1966). It is more in accord with the international anatomical vocabulary. But we shall still talk of the male and female elements of conarticular surfaces. Every pair of conarticular surfaces constitutes a *(synovial) articular unit* (MacConaill, 1973).

Articular Units: Types and Motions

Within one and the same articular capsule there may be one articular unit *(simple joint)* or more than one unit *(compound joint)*. There are 4 types of such units, each of which can be correlated with the *bone-motion(s)* allowed at it. Here we are in the realm of experimental biomechanics, not that of basic motions in the abstract. The 4 types of unit follow.

Using DF to signify degrees of freedom, we have the following types:

1) *Unmodified ovoid* — joints of 3DF; confined to the hip and shoulder joints, both simple.

2) *Modified ovoid* — all other units having ovoid conarticular surfaces.

3) *Unmodified sellar* — units of 2DF whose surfaces are sellar; all have separate articular capsules, although they may form part of bicondylar joints, for example, the temporomandibular.

4) *Modified sellar* — confined to the hinge joints (ginglymi). All have only 1 DF and one separate (simple) joint, except the ulnohumeral.

The association between the types of units and the motions permitted at them is contained in the following statements:

   i) Only unmodified oval units permit pure spin and, therefore, perigyration.

   ii) All units except the modified sellar permit circumduction in both the clockwise and the opposite sense; two further exceptions are given in the next paragraph.

   iii) All units permit arcuate swings that are not part of a revolution; but only the ovoid type permits such swings of both clockwise and anticlockwise kinds from the neutral position.

The pro-supinatory articular units are exceptions to the above rules. All are ovoid but their motions are determined by the binding of the upper and lower parts of the radius to the ulna, so that radial abduction at the radiohumeral joint (unmodified ovoid) is impossible, thus reducing its 3DF to 2DF (swing and spin). This unit is the primary site of pro-supination. The radio-ulnar units (part of a bicondylar joint) are *secondary units*, present because of the need for smooth sliding of the two radial extremities on the ulna, or conversely.

The median atlanto-axial unit is also a secondary joint, the primary sites of motion beween the atlas and axis being the two lateral synovial joints between them (MacConaill, 1973).

In a word, then, *all pivot joints (so-called) are secondary joints*.

REFERENCES

MacConaill, M.A. (1966). The geometry and algebra of articular kinematics. *Bio-Med. Eng.*, *1:* 205-212.

MacConaill, M.A. (1973). A structuro-functional classification of synovial units. *I.J. Med. Sc.*, *142:* 19-26.

FOUR

Composite and Consequential Movements

In anatomical and other medical textbooks muscles are listed as flexors, extensors, abductors and medial or lateral rotators. In our terminology these actions correspond to cardinal swings or to spins. The "textbook way" of describing muscle actions is a useful one for many purposes but it is not always accurate enough, as a simple example shows.

Careful inspection of the terminal phalanx of an index finger shows that in flexion it is supinated (laterally rotated), so that it is brought into a good posture for grasping, say, a needle between itself and the thumb, since the thumb is pronated (rotated ulnarly) in opposition. Correspondingly, this index phalanx is pronated as it moves into full extension. The interphalangeal joint at which these movements take place is rightly called a hinge joint. But the only motions allowed at it are *not chordal but arcuate*, quite unlike those of a carpenter's hinge.

This is one example of a *composite movement*, that is, one in which swing is combined with spin. All hinge joints show this type of motion: all have some degree of rotation combined with flexion or extension. At the elbow, to give another example, the ulna is also pronated in full extension and supinated during flexion.

45

Diadochal and Consequent Motions

At all joints the most common single movements are composite movements, swing and spin together. There is a reason for this. For every joint there is one position in which there is maximal contact between the male and female surfaces of the mating pair; this is the *close-packed position (CCP)*. In this position the articular surfaces are pressed firmly together, and the bones to which they belong cannot be separated by traction across the joint. This is because the chief ligaments of the joint are then in the state of maximal tension; they are not only "tight" but also "taut", like a violin or guitar string that has first been tuned to a particular note and has then been "sharpened". The tightness of the ligaments is brought about by a swing, and they are then made taut by a spin that twists the tightened joint capsule and any extra-capsular ligaments as well. Of course the spin and the swing can be combined in a composite movement and they must be combined at a hinge joint, which has only 1 degree of freedom. It can be shown experimentally that twisting an already tightened articular capsule will cause the articular surfaces to be pressed together, so that the close-packed position is the only one in which ligaments function like muscles.

A table of important close-packed positions will be found at the end of this chapter.

A joint not in its close-packed position (CPP) is in a loose-packed position. Every joint has a *least-packed position* (LPP), in which the capsule is most relaxed (but not the muscles!). For this reason the LPP is very often that of a diseased joint, for it can then accommodate the greatest amount of abnormal fluid in its cavity. A table of least-packed positions will be found at the end of this chapter.

For so long as a joint is in CPP, its bones are very liable to damage by fracture, especially if the CPP is brought about suddenly and violently. For this reason the CPP is normally used only for special effort; though a position very near it is a very common one in all joints, being one in which the congruence (fit) of the conarticular surfaces is almost complete.

Let your upper limb hang vertically downwards, the forearm being in semi-pronation, so that the palm is against the lateral side of the thigh. *Keep the forearm semi-pronated during all that follows*, as if the limb were splinted. Now swing the arm directly forwards and upwards (forward flexion) through 90°, so that it is in a horizontal plane. Next swing it backwards (horizontal extension) through 90°. Lastly, adduct it until it is again hanging down (pendent). Observe that the palm is now facing forwards, that is, *the arm has been rotated through 90° at the shoulder joint*. The forearm is, however, still semi-pronated. Now carry out another 90° of forward flexion, another 90° of horizontal flexion and another 90° of full adduction. Note that the dorsum, not the palm, of the hand is now against the thigh, that is, *the arm has now been rotated laterally through a further 90°*. It will be found impossible to repeat the cycle of movements any further until the arm has been medially rotated at the shoulder through 180°, a fact in accordance with the rule that no bone can be rotated through more than two right angles at any joint.

The "shoulder-swing experiment", as we shall call it, shows us that we can bring about rotation, that is, a spin of the humerus around its long axis, by a succession of movements none of which involves a spin by itself. Forward flexion, horizontal flexion and adduction as carried out in the experiment are all chordal movements, that is, pure swings (cardinal swings). The lateral rotation produced by this succession of swings is, then, a consequence of the succession. Hence it is called a *consequential movement*. This type of movement can occur at any joint having at least 2 degrees of freedom, and is much more common than had been appreciated until fairly recently. How many of those who read this had realised that a simple backward swing of a horizontally held arm brings about a lateral rotation of the humerus?

There is, of course, a law governing the nature and amounts of consequential movements in any given instance. We must first define what is meant by a diadochal movement.

A diadochal movement is the name given to a succession of two or more distinct movements, that is, of movements each of which makes an angle with its predecessor greater than 0° and less than 180°. The name comes from the Greek *diadochos* (successive). Humeral forward flexion (F) followed by horizontal extension (H) is a diadochal movement having two parts, which can be written FH. When we carry out a further movement of adduction (A) we have a diadochal movement of three parts, FHA.

A diadochal movement (DM) may be *open* or *closed*. A closed DM is one that brings the moving bone from and then back to its original position, but, as we have seen, not necessarily back into its original *posture*. If a closed DM brings the bone back into its original posture then it is called an *ergonomic cycle*, because the individual is then ready to start some work-process or other afresh. A perigyration and a circumduction are both ergonomic cycles, although neither is a DM.

The rotation consequent upon a DM is due to the fact that the bones at any joint move through space in curved paths, never in straight lines. This in turn is due to the fact that they move on curved surfaces. The paths of motion lie, of course, on the ovoid of motion. If the path of motion of a bone is along one chord the bone does not rotate, for a chord on an ovoid surface corresponds to a straight line on a flat surface. But as it moves first along one chord and then along a different chord it does rotate, as the shoulder-swing experiment shows. Why? The answer comes from the geometry of ovoid surfaces.

A closed, three-sided figure on any surface is called a *triangle* if and only if all three sides are chords; otherwise it is called a *trigone*. On an ovoid surface *the sum of the three (interior) angles of a triangle is always greater than two right angles*. This is the most important geometrical fact about the kinematics of bones. We shall now state the relevant consequences of it. Rigorous proofs of them will be found in MacConaill (1966); the mathematics involved is strange but easy.

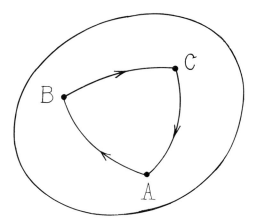

Fig. 4.1. A triangular pathway AB-BC-CA on an ovoid of motion.

Referring to fig. 4.1, if a point on a bone moves along three chordal paths—AB, BC and CA—it will describe a triangle ABC on the ovoid of motion. Let the sum of the angles ABC, BCA and CAB be s. The result of this closed DM will be that the bone comes back to its original position but is rotated through an angle r given by:

$$r = s - 180°$$

The sense of r, clockwise or anticlockwise, will depend upon the sense of the sequence AB-BC-CA: as the sense of the sequence is clockwise or anticlockwise, so is the sense of r. This general statement requires translation into anatomical terms.

In the shoulder-swing experiment the sequence (forward flexion—horizontal extension—adduction) is clockwise for the right upper limb and anticlockwise for the left *as viewed by the subject*, but anticlockwise and clockwise, respectively, *as viewed by an external observer* looking at the subject from in front. From the subject's point of view lateral rotation of the right humerus is clockwise; of the left humerus, anticlockwise. Hence the closed DM defined above results in a

lateral rotation of the humerus. One would expect, then, that
the sequence (abduction—horizontal flexion—extension) would
produce a *medial* rotation, and it does so.

If the path followed by a bone is a triangle, then the consequential rotation takes place during the *second* stage of the
DM, for example, during the passage of the stage BC in fig.
4.1. That is to say, the effect of the "2-leg" DM, along AB
and then BC, is the same as if the bone had first moved along
the path AC and had then been rotated laterally through
the angle *r*. We can write this neatly thus:

$$AB \cdot BC = (AC)E^r$$

in which equation, E^r denotes a lateral rotation through *r*
degrees (or radians, according to the scale of angular measurement used). If, on the other hand, the motion were first along
AC and then along CB, we should write

$$AC \cdot CB = ABE^{-r}$$

since a medial rotation is "negative" if a lateral rotation is to
be taken as "positive".

The rotation consequent upon a DM is a *conjunct rotation*
because it is conjoined with the passage of the bone along the
second side of the triangle ABC (ACB). It is *as if* this chord
were really an arc, passage along which necessarily involved
a spin (rotation) of the bone also.

How large is a conjunct rotation caused by a passage along
the sequence of chords AB-BC? The answer is twofold:

(1) It is as large as the *residual* of the triangle ABC, the residual (*r*) being (*s* − 180°) and *s* being the sum of the interior
angles of ABC.

(2) For one and the same joint, the residual of ABC increases
with the area of ABC, provided that the paths AB and BC
are always traced upon one and the same ovoid of motion.
This is why the difference in area between the male and female surfaces of a joint is a measure of the amount of (angular) motion permitted at the joint, for the greater this dif-

ference, the greater is the amount of swing of the moving bone due to slide.

We must now consider the diadochal movement of a bone along the sides of a *trigone* on the ovoid of motion. In this case one or more of the three sides will be arcs, not chords. Let ABC in fig. 4.2 be a trigone. As in the case of a triangle, the sequence AB-BC-CA will entail a conjunct rotation (r). Again r is ($s - 180°$) if s be the sum of the interior angles of ABC. Indeed, the case of the triangle is merely a special case of the trigone. But in a trigone there is no restriction of the value of s: it may be less than, equal to or greater than two right angles. The cases in which s is precisely 180° are of particular interest. In these instances $r = 0$, and therefore:

$$AB \cdot BC = AC$$

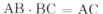

That is to say, the diadochal movement AB-BC is precisely equivalent to the single movement AC, whether AC be an arc or a chord.

From this it follows that if AB and BC be both chords, and if CA be an arc, then the conjunct rotation caused by the sequence AB-BC will be undone by the movement from C to

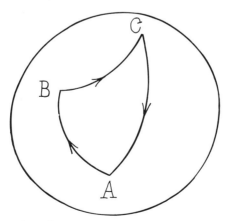

Fig. 4.2. A trigonal pathway on an ovoid of motion. AB and CA are chords; BC is an arc.

A. A closed diadochal movement of this kind is called an *ergonomic cycle* because it brings a limb back into its original position and posture in the course of a repetitive series of work-movements.

All of the paths of motion of a bone could be arcs; indeed this is the usual case, a matter touched upon in the next chapter. Two examples of ergonomic cycles are shown in figs. 19 and 20. In the first of these two of the paths are chords; in the second all are arcs.

Diadochal movements may consist of more than two components if open, of more than three if closed. But no rotation caused by them can exceed that allowed by a maximally rotator arcuate swing: this is a biomechanical restriction. In practice a DM of two or three open paths and ergonomic cycles of three or four paths are all we need to study.

A non-diadochal path, open or closed, is called *monodal* (hodos = path).

The Sites and Prevention of Consequential Motion

Diadochal movements can take place only at joints having at least 2 degrees of freedom, for there is only one possible path of motion at a hinge joint. There is, however, a difference between what is possible at a joint of 2 DF and one of 3 DF.

(1) At a joint of 2 DF the conjunct rotation produced by a DM can be *undone but not prevented*; and it can be undone only by bringing the bone back to its original position. This can be achieved either by traversing the diadochal sequence in the reverse direction (naturally!) or by completing an ergonomic cycle along a single path, usually arcuate.

As an example we can take the movements of a thumb at the first carpometacarpal joint. Let the thumb be in the plane of the palm to begin with and also pressed against it*.

---

* This is the "zero starting position" of the official vocabulary of the American Academy of Orthopaedic Surgeons (*Joint Motion*, 1965). The other terms for motion at the said carpometacarpal joint could be more satisfactory than they are. The terms used here are those found in Cunningham's *Manual of Practical Anatomy*, 13th ed., Vol. 1 (1966).

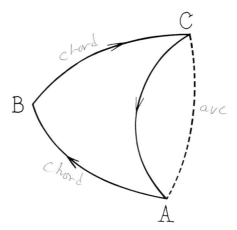

Fig. 4.3. An ergonomic cycle. The sum of the interior angles of the figure ABC (unbroken lines) is 180°. The broken line is the chord of the arc CA. AB and BC are chords.

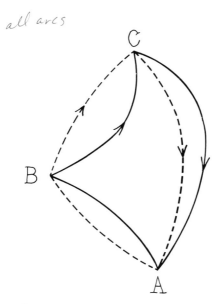

Fig. 4.4. A trigonal ergonomic cycle. Unbroken lines are arcs; broken lines are chords.

Now extend the thumb, *i.e.*, deviate it radially in the plane of the palm. Next abduct it fully from the said plane while still keeping it as much as possible in the extended position. Note that it has come into opposition and has also undergone a pronation around its long axis through about 45°. Finally verify that it can be brought back into its original position and the 45° rotation undone by moving it back along a single path; this path is that along which the thumb could, of course, be brought into opposition by a single movement from its original position, the path of *reposition*.

The sequence (extension-abduction-reposition) clearly constitutes an ergonomic cycle. The path of reposition closes the cycle, and the conjunct rotation consequent upon the first two stages of the diadochal movement (extension-abduction) is gradually undone during the stage of closure.

We can also carry out a four-stage ergonomic cycle with the thumb. In this, the first sequence is (extension-abduction) as before. The second sequence begins with an ulnar deviation of the opposed thumb, kept opposed throughout the movements; note that the pronation of the thumb is maintained. The final stage is again a single movement of reposition, during which the pronation of the thumb is undone. The name "flexion" is given to the first stage of the second sequence, for it is a flexion of the thumb-in-opposition. The whole sequence is, then, (extension-abduction-flexion-reposition).

Using AB, BC and CD to denote extension, abduction and flexion-of-the-thumb-in-opposition, respectively, and using CA and DA to denote the two paths of reposition described above, the reader should verify with the aid of figs. 4.5 and 4.6 that

$$AB \cdot BC = AC \text{ and } AB \cdot BC \cdot CD = AD$$

also that the sum of the interior angles of ACD is 180°.

(2) A joint of 3 DF always permits some independent rotation of a bone moving at it. This rotation is never less than could be carried out by conjunct rotation, but the amount that could be carried out *voluntarily* may be much less. How many

readers who have carried out the shoulder-swing experiment
could rotate their upper limbs voluntarily through even 90°?
And how many were sensible of any rotation during the said
experiment until they had compared the successive positions
of their hands at the end of each cycle?

Nevertheless, it is possible to prevent a conjunct rotation at
a joint of 3 DF by the voluntary use of muscles that can rotate the bone in the sense opposite to the rotation that would
occur otherwise. This is easily shown by a variant of the
shoulder-swing experiment. Again, the forearm and hand
must not be allowed to pronate or supinate.

First put an upper limb in its initial position for the experiment already described. Now *flex the forearm* through a
right angle, *and keep it so* during the new experiment; the
reason for this will be given later. Then flex the bent limb
forwards through 90°. Next carry out a horizontal extension

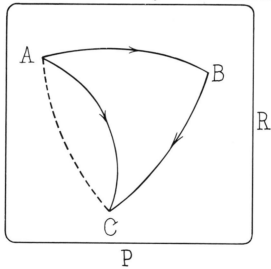

Fig. 4.5. Two paths by which the reader's right thumb can be brought
into opposition; the thumb is viewed from above and a little to the right.
AB, full extension; BC, palmar flexion of the extended thumb, completing
a diadochal path of opposition. AC (unbroken line), single path of opposition; this is an arc to which the broken line is the chord. R and P indicate
the radial and palmar aspects of the hand, respectively.

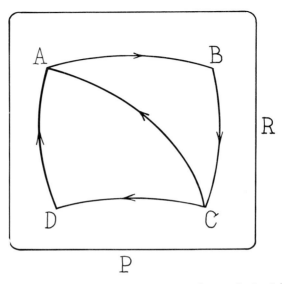

Fig. 4.6. Two diadochal pathways by which the reader's right thumb can be brought first into opposition and then into reposition. AB-BC-CA, trigonal pathway. AB-BC-CD-DC, tetragonal pathway. CA and DA are arcs, all others are chords. R denotes radial side, P denotes palmar side.

through 90°, and also rotate the humerus *medially* through 90° while doing so. Finally adduct the humerus; the limb will come back to its original position and posture. It should then be verified that this cycle can be repeated an indefinite number of times. It is in fact an ergonomic cycle.

Now repeat the experiment with this difference, that the medial rotation of the humerus is carried out during the first stage of the cycle. Observe that at the conclusion of the cycle the forearm points forwards, that is, it has been laterally rotated.

These two experiments prove that the conjunct rotation takes place during the *second* stage of a triangular closed DM, provided that the first stage is a pure swing. Hence the counter-rotation must be applied during that stage if the conjunct rotation is to be *prevented*. The rotation can be *undone* by a counter-rotation applied at the end of the first stage, or in the course of the second stage or at its end.

The reader should also observe that a counter-rotation during the second stage demands more conscious effort, *i.e.*, attention, than does one carried out in the last stage of the cycle. This fact leads to another variant of the experiment, one that explains why the elbow was to be kept flexed during those stages just described.

Carry out the first stage of the original experiment, that is, with the forearm in full extension. Now carry out 90° of horizontal extension, and attempt a medial rotation of the humerus during it. It will be found that the forearm tends to pronate and that, usually, the humerus rotates through only about 45°. If, however, the forearm be deliberately pronated through 90° during this second stage, then the humerus is pronated either only very slightly or not at all; hence the complete cycle can be repeated as often as wished. The significance of this will be considered later.

The Importance of Diadochal Movements

Diadochal movement is much more common than appears at first sight. It is not too much to say that nearly every time an upper limb is used the first motion taken account of is, in fact, the second stage of a DM, for the humerus must be raised (or have been raised) to position the limb for its supposed "first" working motion. Take, for example, a man sliding his hand laterally along a table. He is in fact abducting or adducting a humerus that has already been at least partly flexed forwards. His humerus must, therefore, undergo a lateral conjunct rotation consequent upon the abduction or a medial rotation consequent upon the adduction—*unless counter-rotatory muscles be brought into action to prevent it.* Simple experiments show that this is in fact done if the hand remains on the table or against its edge during the abduction or adduction. For instance, the ergonomic cycle of (partial flexion-abduction-return to knee) can be repeated indefinitely if the hand be raised by the shortest route (chord) from the knee to the edge of the table and brought back to the knee by the shortest route after the chosen degree of abduction has been achieved.

In such cases as the above, specifically rotatory muscles are brought into action as synergists to prevent a conjunct rotation occurring, something that we could not have thought of did we not know about consequential motions.

A very important locus of diadochal movement is the orbit. For example, let a man be looking down at a map. Then let him look upwards at the horizon and then scan it to the right. This is a diadochal movement. During its second stage both eyes will tend to suffer a clockwise rotation about an antero-posterior axis, viewing the eyes from behind. This must be prevented. Hence we find that there are two oblique muscles that can prevent it—the superior oblique for the right eye and the inferior for the left eye. When the head is bent to one side, however, a rotation is allowed to take place, so that the former relation of the retina is allowed as much as possible. Weakness (paresis) or complete paralysis of an oblique muscle is diagnosed by the fact that the retina does rotate in certain movements that are in fact diadochal.

From this brief study of composite and consequential movements we can say that *every muscle is a rotator*, whatever other function it may have. It is an *obligatory* rotator at hinge and pivot joints. At any other kind of joint it is a *potential* rotator, although it may exhibit its rotary power only in the course of a diadochal movement.

The Decomposition of Movements

A diadochal sequence of movements, chordal or arcuate, is equivalent to a single arcuate movement, as we have seen. Conversely, a single movement may be analysed into two or more others, that is, into a diadochal sequence. Thus opposition of a thumb can be analysed into extension followed by abduction.

This *decomposition of movements* is of clinical importance. In many disorders of the central nervous system, notably of the cerebellum, the patient can no longer move a bone from one particular position to another by a single motion but still retains the power to do so by a diadochal motion. There is no need to labour the significance of this for both diagnosis and rehabilitation, as well as for the improved design of artificial limbs.

Note on the Study of Diadochal Movement

It is difficult to understand the theory of diadochal movements and its applications merely by learning rules and looking at diagrams on paper. One needs a three-dimensional model. The best, perhaps, is a sphere painted black, on which lines can be drawn with white or yellow chalk and erased afterwards. Its surface is, of course, an ovoid surface equally curved everywhere. All the theorems in this chapter can be verified on it.

Any part of a meridian of longitude is a chord, as is also any part of the equator. Parallels of latitude are arcs. A rod with a plastic or paper flag can be used for the experiments. It should be slid along chords and/or arcs drawn between points on the sphere. For example, the shoulder-swing experiment can be repeated on the model thus. Starting at the "South Pole", slide the rod along a meridian to the equator, then along the equator for 90° and then back to the pole along another meridian. By marking the course taken with arrows and comparing the first and last positions of the flag on the rod, one can easily demonstrate that the rod suffers a clockwise or anticlockwise rotation as a result of a corresponding sequence of motions on the surface of the sphere.

REFERENCE
MacConaill, M. A. (1966). The geometry and algebra of articular kinematics. *Bio-Med. Eng.*, *1:* 205–212.

Table 1. Close-packed Position of Important Joints

Joint	*Close-packed Position*
Shoulder	Abduction + lateral rotation
Ulno-humeral	Extension
Radiohumeral	Semiflexion + semipronation
Wrist	Dorsiflexion
Metacarpophalangeal (2-5)	Full flexion
Interphalangeal	Extension
1st carpometacarpal	Full opposition
Hip	Extension + medial rotation
Knee	Full extension
Ankle	Dorsiflexion
All toe-joints	Dorsiflexion
All other foot joints	Full supination
Vertebral	Dorsiflexion

Note: Semipronation is the position of maximal congruence (fit) of radio-ulnar joints and of the greatest tension of the interosseous ligament.

Table 2. Least-packed Position of Important Joints

Joint	*Least-packed Position*
Shoulder	Semiabduction
Ulnohumeral	Semiflexion
Radiohumeral	Extension + supination
Wrist	Semiflexion
Metacarpophalangeal (2-5)	Semiflexion + ulnar deviation
Interphalangeal	Semiflexion
First carpometacarpal	Neutral position of thumb
Hip	Semiflexion
Knee	Semiflexion
Ankle	Neutral position
Foot joints	Semipronation
Metatarsodigital	Extension

FIVE

Congruent and Habitual Movements

If we watch ourselves and other folk we find that some kinds of joint movements are associated with others more often than not. Except in those undergoing military or gymnastic training, it is rare to find pure forward and backward swings of an arm except through small angles. It is even rarer (except in a few armies) to see pure forward and backward swinging of the legs—the "Goose Step". Again, a lateral rotation of the forward-swinging arm is more often accompanied by supination than by pronation of the forearm. Indeed, the movement of pronation then requires an effort of attention. These everyday facts lead us to consider what may be called congruent and habitually associated movements. It will be seen that the study of them is a natural sequel to the study of combined and consequential motions made in Chapter 4.

We begin with congruent rotations. *Two rotations are congruent if they are both rotations in the same sense*, though not necessarily at the same rate. Thus, lateral rotation of the humerus and supination of the radius are congruent, for supination is (in the free limb) merely a lateral rotation of the radius around an oblique axis. So also do full extension of the knee and full dorsiflexion of the ankle involve congruent rotations, for the femur rotates medially upon the tibia and the tibia also rotates on the talus. Incidentally, these medial rotations are part of the close-packing mechanisms of the joints mentioned.

The examples just given illustrate the fact that "congruent rotation" is a term applied to the rotation of *bones in series*—humerus-radius, femur-tibia—with respect to the rotations of their shafts. It has a physical significance, as two experiments will show.

(1) Let the upper limb hang by the side of the body, the forearm being fully supinated and the thumb being held loosely against the side of the palm—the "posture of least effort". During the experiment the eyes should be either closed or directed straight forwards. The forearm is then to be pronated as rapidly as possible. In most cases it will be found that the thumb has swung into opposition; that is, it has also become pronated. This pronation of the thumb involves a rotation around its long axis which is congruent with the radial rotation constituting forearm-pronation.

(2) Bring the elbow into full extension, and keep it so throughout the following experiment. Bring the forearm into full supination. Now try to pronate the forearm while rotating the humerus laterally: this will be found to be impossible. Further, it will be found impossible to supinate the forearm and also medially rotate the humerus at the same time. On the other hand, pronation of forearm with medial rotation of humerus or supination of forearm with lateral rotation of humerus are movements easily carried out together.

If, however, the elbow be flexed through a right angle, then any formerly impossible combination becomes possible.

Let us analyse the results of these experiments, remembering that pronation and supination of the elbow are caused by medial and lateral rotation of the radius, respectively. Experiment 1 shows that the angular momentum, *i.e.*, the spin, of the pronating radius is communicated to the thumb, the radius and the thumb being virtually in one line when the *rapid* motion of the radius begins (in slow pronation the thumb does not move away from the palm). The only way the thumb can achieve a pronatory spin is by going into the posture of opposition, and it does so. Muscular effort is required to keep it against the palm in rapid pronation of the forearm.

Turning now to the second experiment, we note that humerus and radius are in one line when the elbow is extended. So long as this co-linearity persists, incongruent rotations of the two bones are not permitted. But they are permitted as soon as flexion destroys the former radiohumeral co-linearity. There is no muscular mechanism to account for the impossibility of incongruent rotations of the two bones with a fully extended elbow: only the biceps and triceps brachii act on both shoulder and elbow joints, and neither can account for the phenomenon. The only other source of the impossibility is in the central nervous system; that is, the cause is *biological*, not mechanical.

Coghill (1929) showed that the developing amphibian body moves as a whole before it moves by parts, and that a developing limb moves as a whole before it moves by parts. He correlated this increasing independence of the parts with the development of the nervous system. His work has since been confirmed and extended to mammals, including man. In their early stages, the radius and humerus are in one line and must both rotate in the same sense if they rotate at all. In the fully developed limb pronation and supination can occur when the elbow is extended and the humerus is not rotating at all, but then no question of incongruent rotation arises. Apparently a reflex inhibitory system is put into operation by the stimuli, leading to lateral or medial humeral rotation of the humerus with the elbow in extension, that is, when the radiohumeral series is in the more "primitive" state. This inhibitory mechanism does not necessarily act when the humerus and radius rotate about different (or non-parallel) axes, as occurs with a flexed elbow.

The name *functional décalage* has been given to the impossibility of simultaneously rotating the radius and humerus in opposite senses when the elbow is fully extended (MacConaill, 1950). The word *décalage* is used by French surgeons to signify the very great reduction of pronation and supination that can take place if the two portions of a fractured radius are not properly re-aligned as part of the treatment of the fracture. When a radius is fractured below the level of insertion of the supinator muscle then this muscle and the biceps brachii supinate the upper fragment of the bone, while the pronator quadratus pronates the lower fragment. In a word, the two fragments undergo *incongruent* rotations. If they are allowed to unite in this new relationship then the upper part of the radius cannot be supinated nor can the lower part be pronated, for each of these movements has already been accomplished! Consequently, the radius cannot rotate at all, or can rotate very little at most.

Every fractured long bone is exposed to the danger of incongruent rotations of its fragments. How this danger is overcome is dealt with in textbooks of orthopaedic surgery.

Congruent Conjunct Motions of a Bone

We have seen in Chapter 4 that a diadochal swing of a bone is equivalent to a single swing together with a conjunct rotation, this rotation being clockwise if the two parts of the diadochal swing form a clockwise sequence and anticlockwise if they form an anticlockwise sequence. That is to say: *The conjunct rotation of a bone is congruent with the diadochal sequence that causes the rotation**.

We can extend the notion of congruence to cover a wider field by saying: *The parts of a diadochal motion and its consequential (conjunct) rotation are congruent with one another and form a "congruent set"*. Take, for example, the shoulder-swing experiment studied in Chapter 4. This showed that flexion (F) followed by horizontal extension (H) is equivalent to abduction (A) together with lateral rotation. Fig. 5.1 shows these motions as they would be seen by the reader looking at a companion's *left* humerus from the left side. In this case

---

* This rule applies to the motions of the bone as traced upon its ovoid of motion, *i.e.*, outside the articular capsule of the joint at which it moves.

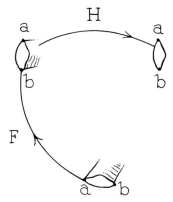

Fig. 5.1. To illustrate the kinematical result of the shoulder-swing experiment described in the text. It shows the displacement of two ints (a and b) on the humerus of the left side after it has been subje..ed to flexion (F), followed by horizontal extension (H). These movements are at the left shoulder and are viewed from the left side. Observe that the bone has been laterally rotated. In each case the movement has been through 90°.

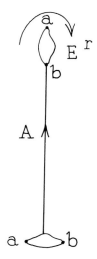

Fig. 5.2. To show the result of abduction (A) through 90° of the same rod as shown in fig. 5.1, followed by lateral rotation (E) also through 90°. Observe that this has the same effect as the previous experiment.

the lateral rotation of the abducted humerus would appear to the reader as a clockwise rotation. As the figure shows, the sequence FH is a clockwise diadochal motion; if we represent the lateral rotation (r) by E^r (the correct way to represent a spin to distinguish it from a swing) then the motions F, H and E^r form a congruent set.

This may seem to be a very abstract way of looking at such concrete things as bone movements. But it provides a clue to the functional interrelation of many movements of a bone (or at a joint) that would otherwise appear to be disconnected. This point will be taken up again later in this chapter when we consider habitual movements. Meanwhile, we proceed to consider another aspect of the congruent set of motions of the humerus that we have just studied, namely, that it enables us to discover two sets of congruent motions of the femur.

Since the humeral sequence FH is equivalent to the sequence AE^r (abduction followed, or accompanied, by lateral rotation), we can write an equation:

$$AE^r = FH$$

This is a "kinematical equation" which summarizes what has been said above about the humerus*. Like other equations in algebra, it can be transformed into several equivalent forms. Before making the transformation we require, it is helpful to recall something we have all learnt at school.

Suppose we have the equation:

$$y = ax$$

Then we can transform this into:

$$y/x = a$$

There is another, often more useful, way of writing the transformed equation, namely:

$$yx^{-1} = a$$

---

* The geometry and algebra of kinematics are fully expounded in MacConaill (1966). This is reproduced in full in Appendix A.

both $1/x$ and x^{-1} being equivalent ways of signifying "the inverse of x".

Now let S represent some swing. Then S^{-1} represents the "inverse motion"—that is, the *reversed* or opposite swing. Similarly, if E^r represents some spin, then E^{-r} represents a spin in the opposite sense. We can now proceed to transform our kinematic equation, bearing in mind that our symbols stand for *kinds* of motion, not for *amounts* of motion (in the present context).

The transformed kinematic equation is

$$F^{-1}A = HE^{-r}$$

It means: Extension (F^{-1}) of a bone followed by abduction (A) is equivalent to a horizontal extension (H) together with (or followed by) a *medial* rotation (E^{-r})—since E^r signifies a lateral rotation.

The transformed equation is easily verified on the upper limb. Point one of your upper limbs directly forwards, so that it is parallel with the ground and the palm is medial. Swing it downwards and backwards without pronating or supinating the forearm. Now abduct it, and note that it is in the same posture as if it had been swung backwards in the horizontal plane and then rotated medially as a whole, *i.e.*, at the shoulder joint. The sequence formed by extension (F^{-1}) and abduction (A) is shown in fig. 5.2 for the left upper limb as seen from the left side, and should be contrasted with the sequence shown in fig. 5.1 for the same limb. As fig. 5.2 shows, the sequence $F^{-1}A$ is clockwise, so that it is congruent with the medial rotation which it causes.

We now turn to the *left* femur as seen from the left side. It is well known that in "full extension" the femur is also abducted and medially rotated to a sensible degree in each case. Our transformed equation will serve for an analysis of the motion of a left femur that is first flexed through a right angle (in a standing subject) and then brought into the position of full extension. It shows that a sequence (*or combination*)

of extension and abduction is enough to account for the observed medial rotation of the femoral shaft, so that the set of
motions constituted by extension, abduction and medial rotation of a femoral shaft is a congruent set.

It follows that flexion, adduction (A^{-1}) and lateral rotation
of a femoral shaft also constitute a congruent set, for we can
transform either our original equation or its transformation
into a third:

$$A^{-1}F = H^{-1}E^r$$

The reader should verify this by reversing the direction of
all the arrowheads in fig. 5.2. He will then understand why
we write $A^{-1}F$ and not FA^{-1} in the above equation.

Now that we understand the meaning of a kinematical
equation it is possible to define congruent sets in a simple
way. If M, N and P form a closed diadochal pathway, if E^q be
a spin, and if

$$MNP = NPM = PMN = E^q$$

then (M, N, E^q), (N, P, E^q) and (P, M, E^q) are all congruent
sets. It should be noted that every such set contains (at
least) two swings and a spin.

Habitual Movements

Opposition and reposition are the most common movements
of a thumb, much more so than extension-flexion or abduction-adduction. The most common movements at the hip joint
are flexion with lateral rotation of the femur and the opposite
motion, extension with medial femoral rotation. Is there, then,
a general rule for determining the habitual motion of a bone?

There is. *The most common movements of a bone are those
that bring it towards or away from the close-packed postion
of the joint at which it moves, along a path passing through
or near to its least-packed position.*

These movements are single movements, that is, not
diadochal. We can call them the "locking" and the "unlocking" movements for short. Every locking movement is the

equivalent of a swing together with a spin. The swing stretches the main ligaments of the joint, and the spin twists its capsule so that the male and female articular surfaces are screwed together. Thus the locking movement must be an arcuate swing, which embodies the rotation due to the spin. This arc is, in turn, the equipollent or equivalent of a pair of pure swings that form a congruent set with the spin. The unlocking movement is, of course, the result of the same arc's being traversed in the reverse direction, so it also embodies a congruent set of motions of the bone.

For example, the hip joint is brought into close-pack by a motion that causes extension, abduction and medial rotation of the femur; we have seen that these are a congruent set of motions. Hence the habitual motions of the femur will be extension with medial rotation and flexion with external rotation. The reader can easily verify that these are the two "natural" ways of swinging a thigh.

Similarly, the first metacarpal is brought into close-pack with the trapezium by the single movement of opposition. This obviously arcuate swing embodies extension, abduction and medial rotation of the metacarpal, the first two motions causing the third if carried out in succession. Here again a congruent set of motions is involved. Opposition and reposition of the thumb are "natural" in a way that flexion-extension and abduction-adduction of the thumb are not. These two latter pairs of movements are used for modifying the basic grasping movement of opposition in what is called the *precision grip* (Napier, 1956). In this grip the first metacarpal is pronated at its carpometacarpal joint, and the first thumb phalanx is also pronated a little at its metacarpophalangeal joint (Napier, 1955). Here we have a pair of serially congruent rotations.

It is to be noted that the posture of the fingers in the precision grip (as in grasping a ball) is one of partial flexion, ulnar deviation and partial supination of all three phalanges. These three movements form a congruent set, for ulnar deviation followed by flexion of a first phalanx at its meta-carpophalangeal (MP) joint will produce supination of the whole finger. The said posture of the fingers, by the way, is an all-too-common permanent result of rheumatoid arthritis of the MP joints.

The other basic form of grip is the *power grip* (Napier, 1956). This is used, for example, for holding the shaft (handle) of a hammer. The four fingers (index to minimus) are the principal agents of this grip, the thumb being ancillary to them if it be used at all. In this grip the MP joints are either in or nearly in their close-packed position—full flexion. The interphalangeal (IP) joints, however, nave moved away from *their* close-packed position—full extension. This difference in the state of the MP and IP joints has a functional meaning. The first phalanges and the palm provide a rigid, or nearly rigid, elongated "female surface" into which the "male" hammer-shaft (or other rod) can fit, while the fingers themselves can be adjusted in their curvature for grasping the "male" object and pressing it against the aforesaid rigid female surface. The reader should carefully peruse Napier's papers cited above for a full account of the power and precision grips and cognate matters.

The Vertebral Column (Backbone)

The vertebral column is a notable locus of habitual movements entailing serially congruent rotations. A book could be written on this important subject alone. What follows here is intended as a guide to the reader's more detailed studies elsewhere.

The suprasacral backbone consists of two major functional parts: the *cervical* and the *thoraco-lumbar*. The cervical part moves the head with its sensory organs in various directions. The thoracolumbar part can twist the trunk and/or increase the forward, downward and lateral range of movements of the upper limbs and head.

About half the total range of motion of the head is due to the cervical part of the column; and it can easily be carried out without any motion of the thoracolumbar part. Motion of the subcervical part can also be carried out without motion in the cervical (to which a nullifying antispin is applied); this is most easily done in a sitting posture and requires practice if it is to be done easily.

Finally, the whole backbone is widely used for conveying the weight of loads carried on the head to the pelvis and lower limb(s) and ground. In this operation the vertebral column is kept in or near its neutral position. This is the biomechanically best way of carrying light or moderate loads; for the weight is borne completely by this part of the skeleton and there is a minimal use of muscle. It also leaves the hands free.

Excepting the first two, every mobile vertebra is attached to the one above it by an intervertebral disc—the occipital bone below the superior nuchal line is a vertebra! The disc would allow every sort of motion of the upper vertebra upon the lower. The function of the pair of synovial joints between two mobile vertebrae is to *limit* motion—most of all in the thoracic segment of the column, less so in the lumbar segment and least of all in the cervical segment, again excepting its atlanto-axial part. Each of these synovial joints can be described as "a structural whole and a functional half". In this they resemble the two temporomandibular joints, for movement at one must be accompanied by a correlative movement at the other. In what follows, the word "joints" will refer to these synovial joints alone; it will not refer to the atlanto-axial or the atlanto-occipital joints unless these be mentioned specifically.

The close-packed position of all the vertebral joints is that of full extension. In this position there is maximal forward convexity of the cervical and lumbar portions of the column, mimimal forward concavity of the thoracic portion and maximal kinking of the lumbosacral junction. It is, of course, rarely assumed. Every joint participates in this mass movement, including the atlanto-occipital, the atlanto-axial and the thoracic set. The momentum of the extending column is transferred *via* the sacrum and sacro-iliac joints to the hip bones (*ossa coxae* or *ossa innominata*). It is not surprising, therefore, that there is a very marked tendency for these bones to move upon the femora and to bring the two hip joints very nearly into close-pack. After all, the only biological purpose served by extreme extension of the backbone in a standing man is to make the eyes look directly upwards.

The anti-close-pack position of the joints is, of course, extreme flexion with minimal convexity of the lumbar portion of the column, maximal forward concavity of the thoracic, definite forward *concavity* of the cervical portion and minimal kinking of the lumbosacral junction. Here again the hip bones tend to share the forward swing of the whole backbone so that the hip joints become somewhat flexed.

The extension and flexion of the backbone provide an example of functional décalage. All know that its cervical part can be flexed and extended without involvement (or, at least, marked involvement) of the lower parts. But *simultaneous* flexion of the neck and extension of the trunk are impossible, as are also simultaneous extension of the neck and flexion of the trunk, *provided that neck and trunk be kept in line with each other*. If, however, the neck be first inclined to the right or the left side then the simultaneous opposite movements of neck and trunk are possible. The reader and a companion should verify this.

The second mass movement of the backbone is best described as *twisting*. It is seen when the head is rotated through 180° in a standing man. Stand upright and turn the head to the right through 90° so that it looks directly to the right. Observe that the whole trunk rotates, as well as the neck. Now turn the head leftwards until it looks directly to the left. Observe that while the neck turns most, yet the trunk also turns for the desired movement of the head to be completed. We can call this whole movement the *complete horizontal* scan*: it involves the whole column. It also involves the hip joints: as the head moves from looking di-

---

* The mass movement from maximal flexion to maximal extension, or contrariwise, can be called the complete vertical scan.

rectly right to looking directly left, so does the right femur become flexed and laterally rotated and the left femur become extended and medially rotated—congruent sets again! In a word, the twist of the vertebral column is transferred in part to an "invisible plate", the visible margins of which are formed by the two femora.

All of the vertebral joints share in the rotation that brings about the horizontal scan. Yet it is quite correct to call the mass movement a twist of the column, for the cervical vertebrae rotate more than do the thoracic and these more than the lumbar. A simple experiment and calculation will prove this. When the trunk is kept facing directly forwards the head can be turned through a total of 90° by a twist of the neck alone. Rotation at each of the 11 thoracic pairs of joints allows of some 5° per joint, giving a total of 55° as their contribution. This leaves 45° to be shared between the lumbar joints and the hip joints.

Horizontal scan provides yet another example of functional décalage. It is impossible to twist the neck to the right and the trunk to the left, or conversely, *simultaneously*. This is so even if the head be first bent to one side. The décalage is probably a safety mechanism, for torsion is the most dangerous *natural* (*i.e.*, "internal") stress that can be applied to a set of bones in series. If one part of the column were to twist to the left and the remaining part to the right at one and the same time, then the torsional stress at the junction of the parts would be equal to the arithmetical sum of the torsional stresses of one of them moving on the other if that other were at rest—just as two automobiles colliding head-on meet each other at a total speed equal to the sum of the speeds of both.

We have dwelt at length upon these two mass movements of the backbone not only because of their actual importance but also because they help us to correct some wrong ideas engendered by the usual statements in textbooks about the movements allowed by the cervical, thoracic and lumbar joints. We shall now give what we think to be. the correct account of these movements in the light of what we know about the contribution of the three sets of joints to vertical and horizontal scanning. It is assumed that the reader has access to a good textbook of anatomy, with text and illustrations he can refer to.

CERVICAL VERTEBRAE. The lower five of these are the most mobile of all the vertebrae. Their joints allow of flexion-extension, abduction-adduction*, rotation about a line behind the vertebral body and a circumduction called "nutation"— like that of a spinning-top in the phase before it comes to rest. Flexion-extension is most marked at the atlanto-occipital joint, rotation at the atlanto-axial. But both these types of motion occur at *all* the joints in a living person, in decreasing measure as the thoracic vertebrae are approached, and all the joints are involved in every type of neck movement. Even the atlanto-occipital joints permit some rotation and abduction-adduction of the head, for their female (atlantal) surfaces are two parts of an incomplete ring upon which one occipital condyle can move forwards and/or sideways while the other moves in the opposite direction.

THORACIC VERTEBRAE. Rotation about a line passing through an intervertebral disk is the *characteristic* motion of a thoracic vertebra, it is clearly not the only one, because these vertebrae share in all the mass movements of the column. It can be carried out without involvement of the cervical vertebrae, but this event demands a marked effort of the will and is not habitual.

LUMBAR VERTEBRAE. Next to the cervical set these are the most mobile. Their joints are so shaped that they permit quite free flexion-extension and abduction-adduction. In daily life, flexion is usually accompanied by some abduction, as when we bend to pick up some object to the right or left below us. This entails a conjunct rotation to the right or to the left, according to the side on which the object is. It is *as if* each lumbar vertebra were first rotated towards the side on which the object is and then inclined downwards towards it by the

---

* Abduction is called "lateral bending" in the English-speaking orthopaedist's vocabulary. Adduction, of course, means the return of the abducted vertebrae towards or to the midline of the backbone.

shortest route. Naturally, the single, arcuate movements that are in fact carried out can take place only when the lumbar joints are in some loose-packed state.

Unlike the cervical joints, the lumbar set have only 2 degrees of freedom, namely, flexion-extension and abduction-adduction. Any rotation at them is always of the conjunct type. As with the other types of movement, all the lumbar vertebrae exhibit conjunct rotation together when we bend this part of the body in order to reach some object that is below and to one side, but the degree of conjunct rotation possible lessens as we pass from the thoracolumbar joint downwards. There is, therefore a twisting of the lumbar column in this operation, just as there is a twisting of the cervical column when it carries out a similar operation, and of the thoracic column also when the whole backbone is engaged, as it usually is.

SCOLIOSIS, LORDOSIS AND KYPHOSIS. These three words come from the Greek and mean (a state of) twisting, concavity and convexity, respectively. They were originally used to describe appearances of a diseased trunk *seen from behind* by the physician, with special reference to the line traced by one of his fingers as he followed the tips of the vertebral spines downwards. The corresponding adjectives are scoliotic, lordotic and kyphotic.

We now know that these three states as described in medical writings are exaggerations of quite normal states. In a man standing upright the cervical and lumbar parts of the backbone are concave backwards—they are lordotic, and the thoracic part is convex backwards—it is kyphotic. When he bends forwards and downwards the lordosis of his lumbar and cervical parts is decreased, the kyphosis of the thoracic part slightly increased. When he bends backwards the cervical and lumbar lordosis is, of course, increased and the thoracic kyphosis very slightly decreased.

Scoliosis is best translated as "coiling", for when a curved rod, particularly a triply-curved rod like the backbone, is twisted it becomes coiled as a simple result of the twist. This is easily verified by applying a twisting force to one end of a piece of wire shaped like the backbone, its other end being held fast. The whole wire becomes coiled around a central axis. The coiling undergone by a normal backbone is like that of a spring that has been lengthened by pulling its ends apart until it nearly, but not quite, forms a straight line.

Natural scoliosis follows a combined flexion and abduction of the vertebral column, particularly of its lumbar part. It is also an accompaniment of a lateral tilting of the pelvis when the neck is kept as vertical as possible or is tilted in the direction opposite to that of the pelvic tilt. It is a "conjunct" movement, following from a set of conjunct rotations of the vertebrae affected. As such it is a simple consequence of the flexion and abduction of the backbone, though it is often stated to be an attempt to maintain the centre of gravity of the body in its position before the pelvic tilt took place. It may well have this effect, but its true genesis is as follows.

Suppose the pelvis to be tilted downwards and to the left (fig. 5.3). Then the longitudinal axis of the first piece of the sacrum will be rotated to the left. This rotation would rotate the whole suprasacral part of the backbone to the left also, a movement that may be permitted by its owner. But usually its owner wants to keep his head vertical. This he does by a muscular pull on the right side of the backbone and ribs from below of such a kind that the thoracic part of the column is pulled to the right. Hence the thoraco-lumbar spine acquires a double curve from side to side: convex to the right above and convex to the left below (fig. 5.4). The thoracic spine has now a double convexity, posteriorly and to the right, and the lumbar spine has now also a double convexity, anteriorly and to the left. This means that the thoraco-lumbar spine becomes coiled, *i.e.*, scoliotic. From below upwards the coil is like that of a piece of wire wound *left-handedly* (anticlockwise) round a thin rod.

In short, a tilt of the pelvis to the left produces a left-handed vertebral coil and a tilt of the pelvis to the right produces a right-handed vertebral coil, tracing the scoliosis *upwards* in each case. These natural scolioses occur when we walk up or down a stairway. They can be exaggerated and become permanent in disease, of the hip

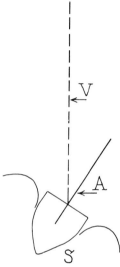

Fig. 5.3. Diagram of a sacrum (S) and neighbouring part of pelvis which have been deviated to the left side from the vertical axis (V). The prolonged long axis of the sacrum is indicated by A.

joint for example. Here we have to do with a normal reaction to an abnormal condition. Whatever our moral habits may be we do try to keep our heads as physically upright as possible!

Movements of the Carpus

We have to distinguish between movements *of* the carpus and movements *within* the carpus. The movements within the carpus are multitudinous and derive their meaning solely from the movements of the whole structure. They could

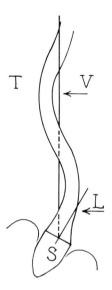

Fig. 5.4. The coiling effect upon the lumbar (L) and thoracic (T) portions of the vertebral column consequent upon the sacral deviation shown in fig. 5.3. The lumbar portion now passes behind the vertical axis (V) while the thoracic passes in front of it. The lumbar and thoracic portions also are bent to the left, and the right, respectively.

be compared roughly with the movements of the balls forming a set of ball-bearings, which are caused by the movements of the part of a machine moving on them. There are, of course, two notable differences between the carpus and a set of ball-bearings: the movements of each carpal bone are quite restricted, and the carpal set of bones comes into and out of close-pack. Indeed, the terms close-pack and loose-pack originated from a study of the carpal mechanism (MacConaill, 1941). Hence the movements of individual carpals will be referred to only when they are of special importance from the clinical aspect. They are caused mainly by forces acting on the metacarpals, or on the radius when the hand is held steady (say, on a table) while the forearm is moved.

Primarily, however, the carpus and metacarpus are to be regarded as a deformable unit, like the vertebral column.

When its ligaments, including the flexor and extensor retinacula, are present this unit is markedly concave on the palmar side near the forearm, less so in its metacarpal part. It is, in fact, arched transversely in diminishing degree as it is followed from forearm to metacarpals. The amount of arching is greatest in full palmar flexion of the wrist, least in full dorsiflexion. This flattening of the arch in carpal dorsiflexion is brought to an end by the flexor retinaculum, which is attached to the most radial-sided and most ulnar-sided bones. It plays the same part with respect to the transverse carpal arch as does the long plantar ligament with respect to the longitudinal arch of the foot*.

The close-packed position of the carpal mass of bones is that of full dorsiflexion, for dorsiflexion converts a relatively loose mass of bones into a rigid mass. Carpal close-pack is brought about in two stages. The first stage is that of extension from the fully flexed position, during which the hand and forearm are brought into one line. In this latter position the hamate, capitate, trapezoid and scaphoid bones are made into a functionally single mass. The second stage is that of full dorsiflexion. The distal carpals *and the scaphoid* move as a whole upon the lunate and triquetrum at the appropriate joints. These joints become close-packed so that the whole carpus is now a functionally single mass, and this mass also becomes close-packed with the radius. Hence *in full dorsiflexion of the wrist the hand and forearm form a rigid mass*. It is then that a fall on the palmar surface of the hand is most likely to cause serious damage—a fracture of lower end of radius (Colles' fracture), a fracture of neck of scaphoid, an anterior dislocation of the lunate bone, etc.

Two facts are to be noted. First, the scaphoid functions, to begin with, as a bone of the proximal carpal row until the hand is extended at the wrist, after which it functions as a bone of the distal row—it "changes sides". This accounts for its

---

* The older (BNA) name for the retinaculum was "transverse carpal ligament". It does in fact serve two functions: it retains the carpal and finger flexor tendons in proper position and it also serves a truly ligamentous purpose upon occasion.

precise disposition in the carpus (fig. 5.5). The reverse is true, of course, as the hand passes from dorsiflexion to palmar flexion. Secondly, the scaphotrapezial joint is unaffected by what happens at the other carpal joints. This reflects the functional independence of the thumb, *for the thumb begins at the scaphotrapezial joint*.

The carpus is, then, divisible into four functional parts, namely:

(A) Trapezium,
(B) Scaphoid,

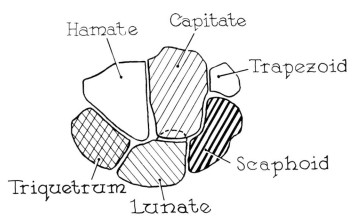

Fig. 5.5. Scheme of the carpal bones mentioned in the text, based on a skiagram.

(C) Hamate, capitate and trapezoid
(D) Triquetrum and lunate.

During the progress from palmar flexion to extension, (B + C) becomes a close-packed set. This set moves on D until (B + C + D) becomes a close-packed set, and itself becomes close-packed with the radius. The set of parts (B + C + D) is that associated with the "power grip" of the fingers, whereas A is associated with the "precision grip" of the thumb and one or more fingers conjointly—as in writing or turning a small screw.

The Big and Little Shoulder Joints

There are really two shoulder joints—the Big and the Little, officially called the glenohumeral and the acromioclavicular, respectively. They work together, for they form part of one mechanical complex (figs. 5.6 and 5.7). This complex consists of the clavicle and certain parts of the scapula: the acromial process, the base of the spine, the glenoid cavity and the base (first part) of the coracoid process (fig. 5.6). It will be recalled that the upper part of the glenoid cavity and the base of the coracoid process are ossified from a cavity so that the big

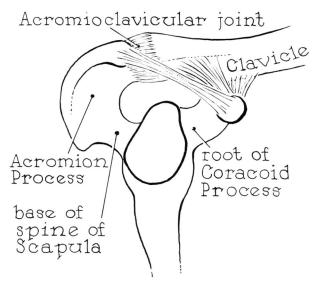

Fig. 5.6. Glenoid cavity (shoulder joint) and acromioclavicular joint, seen from the front. The coracoclavicular ligaments are shown.

shoulder joint is really a scapulo-coraco-humeral joint. The clavicle is linked to the remainder of the complex by the little shoulder joint. At this joint the scapula can swing forwards and backwards, that is, move on the curved chest wall. It can also swing upwards and downwards, this pair of movements being those of greatest extent. Finally, the angle between its upper border and the posterior part of the clavicle can be varied from being somewhat acute to being very nearly a right angle.

When we examine this complex closely, we see that it constitutes a hook, the "shank" of which is the clavicle and the "crook" of which is formed by the remainder (fig. 5.7) Mechanically, the free part of the upper limb corresponds to a weight hung from the hook, as shown in the figure. The acromioclavicular joint (ACJ) is a kind of fracture of the hook, so that crook and shank would come apart in the loose-packed positions of the joint were it not for the trapezius, which

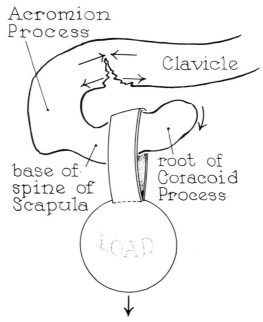

Fig. 5.7. Mechanical scheme of the clavico-scapular "hook". The clavicle forms the "shank" of the "hook" and the scapular components form its "crook". The drawing shows how a heavy weight (*e.g.*, upper limb) acting on the crook tends to "break" the hook. This is prevented by the coraco-clavicular ligaments; compare fig. 5.6.

straddles it and probably helps to hold the clavicle and coracoid process together, being assisted in this by the strong upper ligament of the ACJ.

The close-packed position of the ACJ is brought about by two movements, usually combined. The first of these is an upward and forward swing of the scapula, the second a widening of the angle between scapula and clavicle so that it becomes practically a right angle. These two movements tighten the joint. In particular, the coraco-clavicular ligaments become stretched and tense. As fig. 5.7 shows, they are so placed that they resist the tendency of the shank and crook of the hook to come apart because of the weight of the upper limb carried by the hook.

After the little shoulder joint has been close-packed the upward and forward movement of the scapula is transferred to the clavicle, so that we have the acromial process of the scapula virtually prolonged medially along the clavicle and moving, therefore, at the sternoclavicular joint. Thus the clavicle plays a part in scapular movement like that played by the scaphoid in carpal movement. In the first stage of elevation of the glenoid cavity the clavicle is mechanically a part of the axial (trunk) skeleton, but in the second stage the clavicle "changes sides" and acts as part of the limb skeleton: the parts of the hook are now functioning as a rigid whole. This phenomenon is most marked in abduction of the arm; more correctly, *upward swing* of the same, for abduction properly speaking comes to an end when the arm has been swung outwards and upwards through 90°. During this motion humerus moves on scapula and scapula on clavicle. If the swing of the arm be accompanied by a lateral rotation, then the big shoulder joint comes into close-pack after 90° of swing. The little shoulder joint comes into close-pack during the first 30° of the movement in an unloaded limb, but if the limb be carrying a weight of 5 lbs. (2.25 kg.) this close-packing occurs during the first 10° or thereabouts of scapular rotation on clavicle (MacConaill, 1944).

The Foot

There are some 30 pairs of articulating surfaces in each foot, between which various motions caṅ take place. Fortunately it is not necessary for us to study them in detail, because the foot is divisible into a small set of main parts just like the carpus.

There are three main parts:

(A) The talus,

(B) The subtalar skeleton (*lamina pedis*)

(C) The toes.

Clearly, the "subtalar skeleton" consists of all of the bones not part of (A + C). It is the part whose motions we shall study first. It is used for two main purposes, standing and walking.

STANDING. Mechanically, the subtalar skeleton is a twisted plate that can be untwisted. It is flattened from above downwards along the line of the metatarsal heads. It is flattened from side to side where the heel bone (calcaneus) is, this part being prolonged upwards by the talus. This mechanical schema is shown in fig. 5.8, which shows the twist of the foot-plate (*lamina pedis*) near its maximum. This maximum occurs when we stand on crossed feet. We have near-maximum twist when the feet are uncrossed and side by side (fig. 5.9). Untwisting occurs when the feet are well apart, as is shown in fig. 5.10. This is due to two factors:

(1) The heads of *all* the metatarsals are kept in contact with the ground (through the skin) in *all* positions of standing. (2) The two heel bones are rotated in opposite senses more and more as the feet move further apart (fig. 5.11).

The rotation of the heel bone is conveyed to the other parts of the lamina pedis in decreasing measure as we pass forwards; that is, the foot is untwisted, as can be verified easily upon a foot skeleton with its ligaments intact. Conversely, the feet become more twisted as they come nearer together.

The forms and motions of the joints of the subtalar skeleton can be expressed concisely by saying that they permit the twisting and untwisting of the foot in various positions of standing. This accounts not only for the joints found in the antero-posterior direction but also such medio-lateral joints as those of the sides of the cuneiform bones—at first sight a needless complication!

We now define two terms, pronation and supination of the foot. When the forearm is pronated it is twisted, when it is supinated it is untwisted. So we call twisting of a foot *prona-tion* and untwisting of it *supination*. These terms are to be distinguished from "inversion" and "eversion" of the foot, respectively. The latter two names should be confined to the

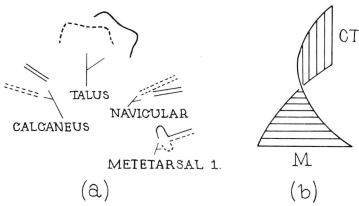

Fig. 5.8. To illustrate the concept of the foot skeleton as a twisted and twistable plate.

(a) Superimposed tracings of rods attached to a right foot in adduction to its fellow (broken outline) and in nearly extreme abduction (solid line); the outline of the upper part of talus is also shown. The rods were placed beside the bones indicated, and the diagram is a tracing from a skiagram taken from in front.

(b) A twisted plate representing the mechanical concept of the subtalar part of a right foot skeleton (*lamina pedis*) viewed from in front as in a. M, line of heads of metatarsals, which do not move during adduction and abduction. CT, vertical axis of calcaneus, which rotates most during twist-ing and untwisting of the lamina pedis. The median plane is indicated.

inward and outward movements of the sole of a foot *when it is off the ground*, these movements taking place mainly at the two joints between the talus and calcaneus. They are cer-tainly not habitual, unlike pronation and supination. Prona-tion involves inversion, and supination involves eversion, but the converse is not true except to a minor extent. If one starts with the back part of the foot in line with the leg, then inversion means that the foot "makes an angle" with the leg on the tibial side, eversion that it makes an angle with the leg on the fibular side. But when the foot is on the ground, then an inward swing of the leg produces not inversion of the foot alone but pronation also, and an outward swing of the leg produces supination as well as eversion.

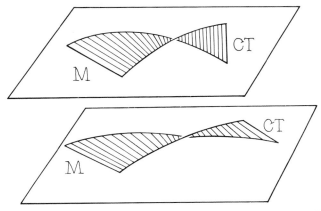

Fig. 5.9. (upper). The right lamina pedis in adduction viewed from the medial side. Observe high, medial longitudinal arch.

Fig. 5.10. (lower). The right lamina pedis in extreme abduction, viewed from the medial side. Observe low, medial longitudinal arch.

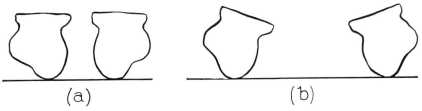

Fig. 5.11. (a) Diagram of right and left calcaneus, seen from behind in adduction. (b) The same, seen in abduction, showing the rotation of these bones.

Supination of the foot is accompanied not only by the rotation of the heel bone around its long axis (fig. 5.11) but also by an outward (lateral) swing of the same bone. In the living subject this is best shown by comparing footprints of the subject taken in three positions: those of pronation, supination and supination combined with dorsiflexion of the ankle (fig. 5.12). As the figure shows, the footprint changes from one like a vertically elongated C to one like an elongated S, the change being due to the outward swing of the heel at the calcaneocuboid joint. If we imagine a recumbent man to be pressing his feet against a vertical board then his calcaneus will be nearly vertical, like the femur and tibia of a standing man. It is then easy to see that the rotation of his calcaneus as his feet pass from the close-together to the wide-apart states is really a *medial* rotation of the bone around its long axis—or, precisely, one congruent with medial rotation of a femur or tibia. Why?

The close-packed position (CPP) of *all* of the joints of the lamina pedis is that of supination of the foot. In the supinated foot, then, the ligaments are most stretched and fully in action, and *in this position alone* can they replace the musculature of the sole of the foot in taking body weight; we shall return to this matter in the next chapter. Conversely, in the pronated foot the ligaments are most lax and least able to replace muscles in maintaining joint posture.

The close-packed position of the ankle joint is that of full

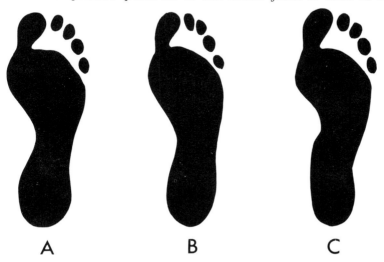

A   B   C

Fig. 5.12. Imprint of a right foot: A, in extreme adduction to its fellow; B, in adduction, the leg being vertical; C, in extreme abduction, the leg being dorsiflexed at the ankle.

dorsiflexion—compare the wrist joint. The attainment of this position involves a small but definite medial rotation of the tibia. This rotation stretches the *anterior* part of the medial collateral ligament and the *posterior* part of the lateral collateral ligament (including the fibulocalcanear ligament). Should full dorsiflexion be brought about violently then the fibulocalcanear ligament may break and we have a "sprained ankle". In many cases this ligament may escape but the stress transmitted by it to the fibular malleolus may cause a fracture of the malleolus, resulting in a "fracture-dislocation" of the ankle—the well-known Pott's fracture. In extreme cases the shaft of the fibula may break; we know of one such mishap that happened to a golfer in Ireland, whose swing was too vigorous for his age!

The ankle joint can be dorsiflexed, of course, whether the subtalar skeleton be pronated or supinated. But when the foot is fully supinated and the ankle is dorsiflexed a special mechanism comes into play. The head of the talus articulates with both the posterior surface of the navicular bone and the upper surface of the sustentaculum tali (on calcaneus). This socket for the talar head lies on the medial side of the subtalar skeleton and has a form remarkably like the acetabulum of the hip bone—whence it has been called the *acetabulum pedis* (MacConaill, 1945). This is certainly a shorter name than the official "naviculo-calcanear surface of talo-calcaneo-navicular articulation"! The acetabulum pedis is shown in fig. 5.13. We can, then, compare the head and neck of the talus to the head and neck of the femur. When the tibia is dorsiflexed on the talus its medial rotation is communicated to that bone. Consequently the head and neck of the talus undergo a rotation congruent with the tibial rotation. This screws the talar head into close-pack with the acetabulum pedis. If the subtalar skeleton is already fully supinated, and so close-packed, then leg, talus and lamina pedis form a close-packed *and rigid* mass of bones.

These facts are of great clinical importance. A fully close-

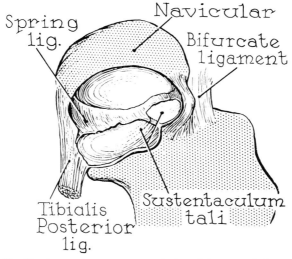

Fig. 5.13. To illustrate the structure of the right acetabulum pedis, seen from above. The inferior calcaneonavicular (spring) ligament is shown passing between the navicular and the sustentaculum tali (which normally has two articular facets as shown).

packed leg-and-foot is specially liable to fracture because of the lack of buffering provided by loose-packed bones. In particular, if a man lands forcibly upon the ground with wide-apart feet and then dorsiflexes his ankles, the torsional moment acting on a talus suddenly brought into close-pack with the acetabulum pedis can bring about a fracture of the talar neck, a fracture comparable with the intracapsular fracture of the femoral neck that is brought about by sudden close-packing of the hip joint. This talar fracture is particularly liable to happen to parachutists who do not obey their instructions to land with feet together. This was a common fracture among paratroopers in the second world war.

There is, then, a remarkable likeness between the working of the forearm-carpus and the leg-tarsus. Each complex is brought into full close-pack by dorsiflexion. Each complex also has a bone that "changes sides". In the extended or plantar-flexed ankle the talus functions as a part of the foot, but in the dorsiflexed ankle it becomes part of the leg for the time being.

The fibula moves upon the lateral side of the talus during pronation and supination of the foot: downwards in supination, upwards in pronation. These movements prevent the development of too great a gap between the fibular malleolus and the talus (MacConaill, 1945). The amount of movement is not large, about 1 mm. or so. But it is important, hence the need for replacing the parts of a fractured fibula and/or tibia in their original position if a good functional result is to be achieved. On the other hand, a damaged foot will function quite well provided it can (1) still bear weight, (2) twist and untwist as required. In any case, some bone could be adequately replaced by fibrous tissue for the fulfilment of the second requirement.

THE ARCHES OF THE FOOT. A lot of sense and also a lot of non-sense have been spoken and written about the "arches of the foot", largely because of a confusion between an "arch" and an "arc". Both words come from the same Latin root (*arcus*), but English allows us to distinguish between them. Every arch is an arc, but not every arc is an arch.

An *arch* consists of three parts: a *keystone* and two "*flanks*", one leading up to the keystone, the other leading down from it. The keystone must be between the flanks of the arch, not above them or below them. Hence the talus does not form part of a "medial arch", for it is above the calcaneus, not between it and the navicular.

There is one true arch of the foot, the so-called lateral arch, a scheme of which is shown in fig. 5.14. It has an ascending flank formed by the calcaneus, a keystone formed by the cuboid bone, and a descending flank formed by the fourth and fifth metatarsals. It elongates somewhat during supination of the foot and, of course, also becomes twisted. The elongation and the twisting are brought to an end mainly by tension in two structures: the long plantar ligament and the abductor digiti minimi muscle below the ligament. This muscle functions

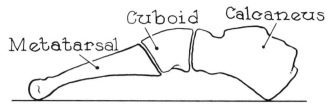

Fig. 5.14. Diagram to show that the lateral arch of a foot is a true arch—calcaneus (ascending flank), cuboid (true keystone) and fourth and fifth metatarsals (descending flank).

more as a ligament than as a muscle, being very fibrous in structure; it contrasts markedly with the very fleshy abductor hallucis.

In supination the lateral arch is lowered; in pronation it is heightened. So long as a foot has a lateral arch it is *not* a "flat foot". The lamina pedis is properly described as a *curved*, twistable and untwistable plate, the basic curvature being that of the lateral arch.

In contrast, the so-called "medial arch" is the result of the twist that brings about pronation, and is markedly lowered by supination. In long feet it is lower than in short feet, a fact to be borne in mind when one interprets a single footprint of one foot. Of course, single footprints should never be taken. Footprints should be taken of both feet in *three* positions: when close together and when wide apart, both with legs vertical; and when wide apart with the ankles dorsiflexed. If the kinds of changes shown in fig. 5.12 are seen, then the feet are functionally not flat feet.

WALKING. Normal walking is best studied on a single foot raised from the ground, which undergoes the following cycle of motion:

(1) It is thrust forwards and downwards until the *heel* touches the ground.

(2) It is then swung downwards so that the *lateral arch* is in contact with the ground at its extremities.

(3) It is then *semisupinated* so that there is maximal contact between the sole and the ground.

(4) It is then *fully supinated* and the heel is raised off the ground in such a way that the thrust is transferred to the ball of the big toe and the first metatarsophalangeal joint is dorsiflexed.

(5) Finally the said joint is straightened and the foot is raised upwards and backwards from the ground. The foot becomes pronated while it is off the ground.

The reader should walk slowly—like a mannequin—and verify that the above cycle occurs, also that stage 4 in one foot is synchronous with stage 2 in the other foot. It should also be verified that any other cycle gives an abnormal gait.

Broadly speaking, the later phase of walking results in the transference of full body weight from one, pronated foot to the other, supinated foot.

Again, the main upward pull of the plantar-flexor muscles of the ankle upon the heel occurs when the foot is close-packed or nearly so. The rising foot then becomes more loose-packed.

If possible, the reader should experiment upon an osteo-ligamentous preparation of the leg and foot, the femur having been removed from the knee joint. In most cases this will remain stable upon a table top if the leg bones are vertical. If these bones are now pushed directly forwards the ankle will become dorsiflexed. If the forward push be continued stages 2-4 of the walking cycle will occur automatically.

These experiments help to establish the following points:

(1) Gravity alone can bring about supination of the foot (flatter arch).

(2) Muscles acting on the plantar part of the foot are required for pronation (higher arch).

(3) The weight of the body together with a forward thrust upon the tibia at its upper end is enough to bring the weight of the body to bear, first upon the lateral arch and later upon the ball of the big toe, and also to raise the heel a little.

(4) All other parts of the cycle of walking require muscular force.

REFERENCES

Coghill, G.E. (1929). Early development of behaviour in amblystoma and in man. *Arch. Neurol. and Psychiat.*, *21:* 989-1009.

MacConaill, M.A. (1941). The mechanical anatomy of the carpus and its bearings on some surgical problems. *J. Anat.*, *75:* 166-175.

MacConaill, M.A. (1944). The mechanical anatomy of the acromio-clavicular joint of man. *Proc. Roy. Irish Acad.*, Sect. B, No. 7, 159-166.

MacConaill, M.A. (1945). The postural mechanism of the human foot. *Proc. Roy. Irish Acad.*, Sect. B, No. 14, 205-278.

MacConaill, M.A. (1950). Rotary movements and functional décalage. *Brit. J. Phys. Med.*, *13:* 50-56.

MacConaill, M.A. (1966). The geometry and algebra of articular kinematics. *Bio-Med. Eng.*, *1:* 205-212.

Napier, J.R. (1955). The form and function of the carpo-metacarpal joint of the thumb. *J. Anat.*, *89:* 362-369.

Napier, J.R. (1956). The prehensile movements of the human hand. *J Bone and Joint Surg.*, *38B:* 902-913.

SIX

The Potential Actions of Muscles: Kinematic

Every skeletal muscle has two functions. One is to swing and/or spin a bone through some range of angles; the other, often forgotten by kinesiologists, is to provide the whole body with a substantial part of its necessary heat. The first of these functions is to be studied under two aspects, the kinematic and the kinetic, so that we can talk of myokinematics and myokinetics.

Myokinematics has to do with the way in which the structure and arrangement of a set of muscle fibres determines the *amount* of angular motion associated with its full contraction, and so the range of movement it can help to occur.

Myokinetics deals with the *forces* required to make the kinematic properties of muscles effective, with the part played by gravity in this affair, with the selection of muscles for particular tasks. It will be dealt with in Chapter 7. In this one only myokinematics is considered.

The Two Laws of Myokinematics

A muscle produces its kinematic effects in one or both of two ways, by *Approximation* or by *Detorsion*. Approximation refers to the bone(s) acted upon, detorsion to the muscle itself. These effects can be expressed in the form of two laws, whose operation can be demonstrated on a simple apparatus called a Psalloscope (MacConaill, 1973)*.

---

*The article referred to contains full instructions for making the apparatus, together with photographs illustrating its parts and their uses.

95

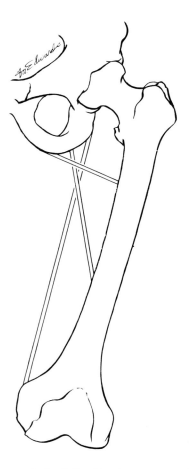

Fig. 6.1. Three myonemes of the left adductor magnus. In this case they are part of a twisted muscle.

Law of Approximation. When a muscle contracts it tends to bring its attachments (origin and insertion) closer together. This scarcely needs proof!

Law of Detorsion. When a muscle contracts it tends to bring its line of origin and its line of insertion into one and the same plane.

The law of detorsion applies, of course, only to muscles that are *twisted* in some measure at the beginning of contraction. The typical example is the sternomastoid. When an upright man is looking directly forwards the origin of, say, his *left* sternomastoid is along a line running from right to left; its insertion is along a line running from front to back on the side of his skull. It is clearly a twisted muscle. By the law of approximation it can bring the side of his head nearer to his shoulder girdle. By the law of detorsion it can swing its line of insertion into the same plane as its line of origin, that is, turn his head to the right. Its complete action, therefore, will be to bring his *left* eye into the position of that of a hen looking at a nice, fat worm!

There are many more twisted muscles than appear at first sight. One such is the *adductor magnus*. Its fibres pass laterally to the femur from an antero-posterior line of origin along the lower margin (conjoined ramus) of the hip bone to a supero-inferior insertion on the femur. By the law of approximation it is an adductor and also an *internal* rotator of the hip, for its line of insertion is behind the long axis of the femur and the two actions named will bring its origin and insertion closer together. Its fibres are so arranged that the law of detorsion makes it a potential extensor of the hip should the muscle act as a whole. Another twisted muscle, one of great importance, is the clavicular head of the pectoralis major. Its line of origin is horizontal in an upright man; its insertion is vertical when his arm is hanging downwards. Clearly, flexion of the humerus at the shoulder brings the two lines into one plane; it has long been known clinically, and has been verified by electromyography, that this muscle is the chief flexor for the (big) shoulder joint, a function not obvious to the eye because of the oblique course of the muscle fibres towards the humerus.

The function of many muscles can be well understood when it is realised that they are made to twist because of some normal movement. In a standing man the chief, that is *sacral* line of origin of the gluteus maximus is in the same plane as the femoral insertion of the muscle. But if he bends his trunk forwards then its origin becomes horizontal; that is, flexion at the hip twists the muscle. Hence gluteus maximus is a powerful extensor of the hip, particularly when acting on a forward-bent trunk, a conclusion that has been verified by electromyography.

Connected with the topic of twisted muscles ‘is that of *cruciate muscles.* This name is applied to muscles that have parts that cross each other in the form of an X. There are many cruciate muscles. The sternomastoid is not only twisted but also cruciate. Its official name is "sterno-cleido-mastoid" but it is more truly designated as *sterno-occipito-cleido-mastoid.* Its sterno-occipital and cleido-mastoid (claviculo-mastoid) parts cross each other in X-fashion and are easily separated by a dissector's finger. The adductor magnus is also cruciate, for its upper, pubofemoral fibres are nearly horizontal and lie in a plane anterior to that of the more vertical, ischiofemoral set. Indeed, the pubofemoral part is often reckoned a separate muscle and called "adductor minimus." Finally, the clavicular head of pectoralis major is very much a cruciate muscle: those fibres originating medially from the clavicle are inserted into the humerus higher than are those originating laterally.

All cruciate muscles become twisted (or more twisted) by a movement opposite to that which they cause *when acting as a whole.*

Muscle Fibres, Myones and Myonemes

Every skeletal muscle can be analyzed into three kinds of units: structural, contractile and kinematic. The latter two have, of course, structural units as a basis. The structural unit is called a *muscle fibre;* the contractile, a *myone;* and the kinematic, a *myoneme.*

Muscle Fibres. These are really the elongated multinucleate cells of which every skeletal muscle is composed and from which its properties proceed. The term "fibre" is an unfortunate one, but it cannot be abandoned at present.

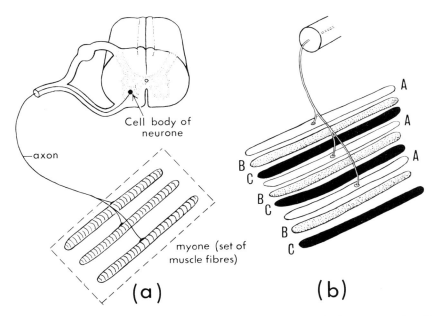

Fig. 6.2. (a) Diagram of a motor unit; it is composed of a neuronal cell body, its axon and the myone it supplies. (b) Myones intermingle and occupy neighboring fasciculi; here fibres of three myones — black, gray and white — are shown diagrammatically within a small part of a muscle.

Myones. A myone consists of a set of muscle fibres that are all innervated by one and the same motor nerve and by no other. The fibres of one myone are found among those of neighbouring myones, so that these contractile units are distinguished by innervation, not by position within the muscle, from each other. See fig. 6.2.

It follows that the contractile units of a muscle are not its fibres but its myones, for each myone must contract as a whole because of its innervation. It has been found possible to elicit the contraction of single myones in trained subjects (Basmajian, 1963); this implies that motor neurones can also be brought into action singly, thus verifying Sherrington's concept of neuromuscular units. "Myone" is a shorter word for such a unit; it could also be called a "neuromyone."

Because of the intermingling of neighbouring myones, one or more myones can go out of action while an equal number of "overlapping" myones takes their place without changing the direction or strength of the muscle-pull. This permits *shift-work* (ouvrage tour-à-tour) within a muscle when it is not exerting its full strength.

Myonemes. A myoneme is the thing called a "muscle fasciculus" in anatomical textbooks. It consists of a bundle (fasciculus) of muscle fibres and, therefore, myones together with any associated tendon; and it passes from a "bone of origin" to a "bone of insertion." Most myonemes pass over the joint(s) on which they act, but there are exceptions; these include the vertebro-scapular, the intercostal and the abdominal wall muscles. Adductor magnus myonemes are shown in fig. 6.1.

Myonemes are the kinematic units of muscle, for the amount of movement of a bone (measured in angles) is wholly dependent upon the contraction of the active muscles(s). This contraction (shortening) can be complete or partial, depending upon the number of myones-in-series acting. Complete shortening will cause a swing of $A°$ and a spin of $R°$, so that associated with every myoneme there are two *kinematic ranges,* namely, $0-A°$ and $0-R°$. The factors determining this range have been studied in detail by MacConaill (1971); and much of this chapter is based upon the results of that study.*

The contractile part of every myoneme consists of myones, though it may share some of these with other myonemes (Sissons, 1969). This has two consequences:

i) The *speed* with which a myoneme contracts is the speed with which its individual motor neurones come into action, and is therefore determined by the nervous system.

ii) The contraction of every myoneme is *saltatory* ("by jumps") although this is masked by the visco-elastic effect of

---

*The article cited is a mathematical development of simple, well known myological facts.

the myonemes themselves and of the connective tissue around them.

These two conclusions apply, of course, to the muscles of which the myonemes are part.

It is this neural control of speed that makes both slow and small movements possible at will. Infants are jerky. The art of slow, graceful movement takes time and effort to learn, reaching its summit in such people as the great ballerina and the skilled craftsman. As we shall see, the structural modifications of myonemes are for lessening, not increasing, the range of movements they produce.

Types of Myonemes. A myoneme may consist wholly of contractile parts or may have tendon at one or both ends. The first type is a "holomyoneme", the second is a 'tendomyoneme" (MacConaill, 1971). However, as these two terms are rather long, we shall call the first type a *holoneme* and the second a *tendoneme. Note:* — the word *nema* is Greek for "string" or "fibre." By using it we avoid the confusion caused by using the Latin *fibra.* English allows this distinction!

Structural Types of Muscles. Muscles can be classed as either *holonemic* or *tendonemic,* the second being by far the most common; these names explain themselves.

There are two kinds of tendonemic muscles, the *collinear* and the *pennate.* In the collinear kind the contractile and the tendinous parts are in one and the same line. In the pennate kind the contractile parts join the tendon obliquely, although some pennate muscles have a collinear part also. The tendon of a pennate muscle is formed by the fusion of the successive tendinous parts of its tendonemes.

Functional types of myonemes and muscles. A myoneme or muscle can be of one, but only one, of three types: *chordovial, gyrovial* or *arcuvial.* The suffix *-vialis* means in Latin "type of path."

A chordovial myoneme produces a pure (cardinal) swing, that is one along a chordal path in space. A gyrovial myoneme produces a pure spin (compare "gyroscope"). An arcuvial myoneme produces both swing and spin as the result of its total contraction. For "myoneme" we can put "muscle" in each case.

Although there is only one chordovial and one gyrovial muscle on each side of the body, yet the study of chordovial and gyrovial kinematics help us to understand all myokinematics, because the action of an arcuvial muscle can be analyzed into chordovial and gyrovial parts. Moreover, it will be shown that the conclusions reached by MacConaill (1971) for pure swing muscles are applicable to spin muscles also. Hence these conclusions will be stated (not proved) and applied to the other types of myonemes after that.

Before stating these conclusions we recall an experimental fact: *no spin or swing of a bone at a joint can ever exceed 180°*. This is the Law of Restriction (of uniarticular movement).

We also recall that *every bone moves at some articular unit* — Law of Location (of movement). This law holds even for the scapula. What are called "rotations" and "translations" of this bone are really the result of swings at the acromioclavicular joint and/or movements of the clavicle at the sternoclavicular joint; a statement easily verified by the reader.

Chordovial Kinematics

Let a chordovial myoneme arise from a bone at a distance c from the axis around which it helps to swing the other bone of an articular unit; let it be inserted into that other bone at a distance q from the said axis; let it have a proportion of tendon t; and let A be the angle associated with its maximal contraction. Then A is determined completely by two ratios. One of these is t. The other ratio is p, which is c/q; it is called the *partition-ratio*, because it is the ratio of the two parts of the sum $(c+q)$.

Let the reader look at fig. 6.3. In each of its diagrams M is a myoneme. The distances c and q are called the *cisarticular* and *transarticular* lengths, respectively. These distances are

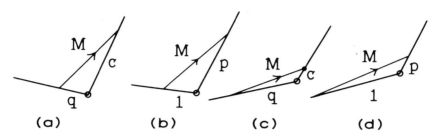

Fig. 6.3. To illustrate the concepts of the cisarticular length *(c)*, the trans-articular length *(q)* and the partition-ratio *(p)* associated with a myoneme *(m)*. In (a) and (b) $p > 1$; in (c) and (d) $p < 1$. See text.

constant for any one myoneme, so that we can take q as the unit of measurement for all lengths associated with that myo-neme. Thus c and q can be replaced by p and 1 in calcula-tions. (This is shown in figs. 6.3b and 6.3d.) Lastly, if any two myonemes are parallel to each other, then p is the same for each, as was shown by Euclid long ago; and this will be true for *all* stages of their contraction, since c/q is always constant for each myoneme.

We next consider the difference between two particular lengths *of any myoneme whatsoever*. One of these is s, the length of a normally fully stretched myoneme. The other is z, the length of the fully contracted myoneme. The "contractile length" of s is obviously $s(1-t)$, so that z is $s(1+t)/2$ (Mac-Conaill, 1971). Hence:

$$z/s = (1+t)/2 \text{ and } s = 2z/(1+t)$$

The equation for z/s is the biomechanical foundation for all myokinematics and should be remembered. It was shown in the article mentioned above that the essential conclusions we shall find are not altered by taking z/s to be as high as $(3+2t)/5$ or as low as $(2+3t)/5$.

We now consider the equations for flexor and for extensor myonemes. These equations do not give the value of A but of $\sin^2 A/2$*. However, because of the Law of Restriction, $A/2$

*Expressions like $\sin^2 A/2$ are to be read as if written $\sin^2(A/2)$.

can never exceed 90°, so that if we know $sin^2A/2$ then $A/2$ (and hence A) can be found unequivocally from a table of square roots (or squares) and from a table of sines — or directly from a computer. In particular, if $sin^2A/2$ take the successive values ¼, ½, ¾ and 1, so does A take the corresponding values 60°, 90°, 120° and 180°. These numerical values are enough for our purposes.

$\gamma = 180° - A$
Law of Reciprocation

$Sin^2\left(\dfrac{A}{2}\right)$ cannot > 90 (never)
Law of restriction

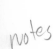

Fig. 6.4. A fully contracted flexor chordovial myoneme associated with a swing of $A°$ from extension of the mobile bone. See text.

We now look at flexor (collinear) myonemes. Remember the substitution of p and 1 for c and q, let the flexor myoneme be of length $(p+1)$ when fully stretched in extension as in fig. 6.4. Then let it contract fully so that its length becomes z when it has swung the mobile bone through an angle A. As the figure shows, z is now the base of a triangle whose other sides are p and 1, and whose apical angle is $(180°-A)$. Since z is $(p+1)/(1+t)/2$, we find from trigonometry that:

$$sin^2A/2 = \frac{(p+1)^2\,(3+t)\,(1-t)}{16p}$$

This is the *kinematic equation for chordovial flexors.*

notes

Thus, if $p = 1$ and $t = 0$ then $sin^2A/2 = 3/4$ and $A = 120°$. Again, if $p = 3$ and $t = 1/5$ then $sin^2A/2 = 64/75$ and $A = 137°$. Again, if $p = 3$ and $t = 1/5$ then $sin^2A/2 = 1$ and $A = 180°$. Thus the effect of tendon is to reduce the kinematic effect of a muscle with a given p.

From this equation we derive five important conclusions now to be stated. The reader can verify them easily:

i) Range of motion $(0-A°)$ proper to a flexor myoneme acting on one joint is determined wholly by its partition-ratio and the proportion of tendon in it; that is, by its p and t, not by its absolute length.

This gives a functional meaning to the distances of the origin and of the insertion of a flexor muscle from the axis of motion of the articular unit on which it acts.

ii) The said range of motion is unaltered by reversing the direction of pull of the muscle.

This is because the value of t is unchanged as also is that of $sin^2A/2$ when $1/p$ (= q/c) is substituted for p, the new partition-ratio being $1/p$ because functional origin and insertion are reversed.

iii) The p of flexor holonemes must lie within the limits 1/3 to 3; and these all cause large swings.

This surprising conclusion is proved by putting $t = 0$ and $p = 3$, as was done in one of the numerical examples above; A is then $180°$. But it is a biomechanical fact that no swing of a bone at an articular unit is ever as much as $180°$, not even at the elbow and hip (where the range is 0-144°); this proves the first part of the conclusion, independently of the Law of Restriction. The second part follows from the equation itself.

iv) *Myonemes must be tendonemes* if p is outside the limits 1/3 to 3; but they *can* be tendonemes even within these limits.

This is a corollary of (iii) above.

v) *The primary function of tendon is kinematic;* it is essential for keeping the motion caused by myonemes of large p within the range of motion permitted by the surfaces, capsules and ligaments of the joints on which they act. This follows immediately from (iii).

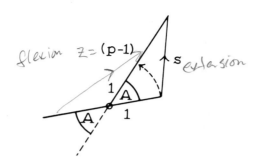

Fig. 6.5. A fully stretched extensor chordovial myoneme about to restore full extension after flexion of the mobile bone through $A°$.

We now turn to *extensor* myonemes, those whose full con-traction completely undoes a previous flexion of a bone through a full flexion of $A°$, and have been fully stretched by that flexion.

The reader should look at fig. 6.5. It shows an extensor myoneme whose partition-ratio is p, and which has been stretched to its full extent s by previous flexion of the mobile bone through the angle A. This time we have an initial tri-angle, whose sides are s, p and 1, with an apical angle A. When fully contracted the myoneme becomes of length $(p-1)$; that is $z = (p-1)$; as the reader should verify, using the fact that the myoneme and the bone on which it acts are then in one straight line. We have, therefore, $s = 2z/(1+t) = 2(p-1)/(1+t)$. From trigonometry we then find:

$$sin^2 A/2 = \frac{(p-1)^2\,(3+t)(1-t)}{4p(1+t)^2}$$

This is the *kinematic equation for chordovial extensors*. It is more complex than that for flexors; but both are, in fact, forms of the single equation for all chordovial muscles: $(s^2-z^2) = 4p \sin^2 A/2$.

This equation clearly excludes the value $p = 1$. Again, when $p = 3$ and $t = 0$ then $\sin^2 A/2 = 180°$, so that extensor holonemes, like flexor, must lie within the p-range 1/3–3 (with a break at $p = 1$). It follows that the set of conclusions drawn from the flexor kinematic equation also holds for extensor chordovial myonemes. We can go one important step further, however.

Since $\sin^2 A/2$ must be less than 1 — an anatomical, not a purely mathematical fact — we can find from either of the two kinematic equations that value of t which *must be exceeded* if p has any assigned value. This is done by first putting $\sin^2 A/2 = 1$ and then solving the equation for t in terms of p; then t must be greater than the value found in this way. Doing this, we find the *t-inequality* (as it is called technically):

$$t > \frac{p-3}{p+1}$$

Thus as p takes the successive values 4, 7 and 11, so must t be greater than 1/5, 1/2 and 3/4, respectively. The increase of t with that of p becomes less and less as p increases. When $p < 1$ then $1/p$ is substituted for p in the equality; that is, the myoneme is measured from its anatomical insertion, not from its anatomical origin.

There is also a p-inequality, which follows from the t-equality, as is easily verified. It is:

$$p < \frac{3+t}{1-t}$$

Thus if $t = 1/2$, $p < 7$, as we already have seen.

At most joints, however, the swing from extension, or even the total swing, does not exceed 90°. For this angle $\sin^2 A/2 = 1/2$; using this value instead of 1 in either kinematic equation we find:

$$t > \frac{p\text{-}1}{p\text{+}1}$$

Hence for the p-values, 4, 7 and 11 we find that t must be greater than 3/5, 3/4 and 5/6, respectively; a very considerable increase in t compared with the values found earlier.

In particular, as p approaches 30, so does t approach 29/31, that is, 93 per cent of the myoneme length; and for $p = 59$, $t > 97$ per cent! In the latter case, the contractile part of the myoneme would be less than 3 per cent; so that if a myoneme were 30 cm long it could contract through less than 5 mm, an absurdly small amount. These figures are, of course, for *collinear* muscles. An arcuvial muscle must have an even more efficient contractile power. How the difficulty of combined great p and small A is solved will be shown when we come to pennate muscles.

Meanwhile we note that our study of collinear chordovial myonemes has revealed that the structure and function of myonemes, therefore, of muscles also, are related in a numerically expressive way.

Before considering gyrovial muscles we look at the only chordovial muscle in the body.

Pronator quadratus: This muscle (fig. 6.6) acts by swinging the lower third of the radius around an axis passing downwards through the head of the ulna — the "oblique axis" of the textbooks is a purely mathematical construction. Its myonemes pass transversely, or nearly so, across the vertical axis defined above to their insertions on the body of the radius. The p of the longest myonemes approaches 3, according to the range of pronation which is 0-180° (very nearly), for all but the lowest of them are holomyonemic. It is, in fact, an ideal swing muscle.

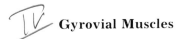

Gyrovial Muscles

There is only one gyrovial muscle on each side of the body, namely, the ulnar part of the supinator. The pronator teres is

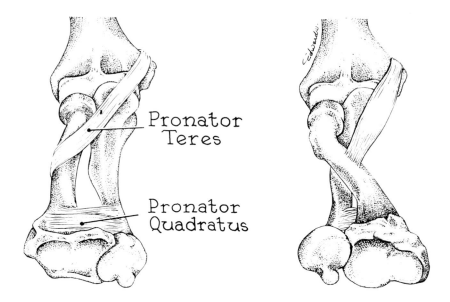

Pronator
Teres

Pronator
Quadratus

Fig. 6.6. A chordovial muscle (pronator quadratus) and an arcuvial muscle (pronator teres) and their effects on the radius in pronation.

arcuvial, being a flexor-pronator.* A study of the supinator is a necessary prelude to that of arcuvial muscles.

Every myoneme of the (ulno-radial) supinator is fully stretched when the radius is fully pronated. In this state the myoneme is wrapped (wound) around the radius from above downwards so that it forms part of a helix ("spiral") (fig. 6.7). The part of the radius involved is practically a cylinder of circular transverse section, with a long axis in its middle running upwards to the capitulum of the humerus; and pronation and supination of the *upper* part of radius are spins around this axis.

If a supinator myoneme passed transversely around part of

---

*Gyrovial muscles and arcuvial muscles were called "monokinetic" and "polykinetic," respectively, in the first edition. The present names are more exact.

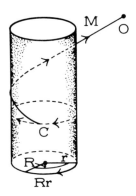

Fig. 6.7. Diagram of a gyrovial myoneme (M) before rotation starts. O: origin of myoneme. C: circle of insertion. r: radius of C. R: angle of rotation associated with full contraction of M.

the radius its part on the radius would be part of a circular line (fig. 6.8); use will be made of this mathematical fact later. But it actually passes obliquely (spirally) round the bone; hence, when it contracts its insertion-point will be moved upwards around the above-mentioned radial axis along an *elliptical* line, as geometry tells us. Calculations involving such lines would require the use of "elliptic integrals." These are trifles for computers but not for ordinary folk; even mathematicians in general dislike them! Happily,

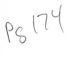

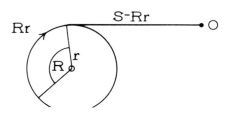

Fig. 6.8. A gyrovial myoneme passing transversely across the mobile bone and of initial length *s*. Other symbols as in fig. 6.7.

we can obtain such information as we need for our present purposes by considering the hypothetical case in which a myoneme passes transversely around the radius (fig. 6.8).

As the figure shows, four quantities are involved in this simple case: a myoneme of length s, of which a proportion t is tendon; a bone whose transverse section is of radius r; and an angle R, through which the full contraction of $s(1-t)$ spins the bone. This requires that the insertion of the bone should move along the circular arc Rr. We have, therefore:

$$\frac{s(1-t)}{2} = Rr \text{ and } R = \frac{s(1-t)}{2r}$$

In this equation R is expressed in *radians*; it will be recalled that 3.14 radians = 180°, so that 3 radians is 173°.

For a given R and r, a holoneme in this case would be of length $2\ Rr$ when fully stretched; for all of its contraction would be effective in rotating the radius, since the two radio-ulnar joints prevent any swing in any direction. On the other hand, if the myoneme were parallel with the radius it would produce no rotation whatever. It is clear from these two facts that the less transverse the myoneme the less will the effect of its contraction be; so that it must be longer than a transverse myoneme of the same structure to help to produce the rotation R. Hence for helical myonemes,

$$s > \frac{2\ Rr}{s\ (1 - t)}$$

In the case of the supinator of an adult r = 0.5 cm and R = 3 = 173° in typical instances. It follows that s = 3 cm. The longest (and superficial) ulno-radial myonemes are more vertical than horizontal and so must be much longer than 3 cm. They are, in fact, 6 cm long or thereabouts. It is *as if* they were transverse tendonemes having t = 1/2 and of length 6 cm at the start of supination.

Arcuvial Muscles

There are three classes of arcuvial muscles:

i) Those which always produce arcuate motion;
ii) Those which can produce chordal motion as well as
   arcuate, if suitable other muscles come into action to prevent the conjunct rotation that would otherwise occur;
iii) Those which can produce pure spin, and pure swing as
   well as arcuate swing, again if suitable other muscles act
   with them.

The first class acts upon hinge-joints (ginglymi); examples
are brachialis, flexores digitorum and the lumbricals.

The second class acts upon joints of 2 degrees of freedom.
The biceps brachii and interossei are examples.

The third type acts upon the hip and shoulder joints; and
upon the vertebral column (including the head) which is a
chain of joints (articular chain, *Gelenkkette*) acting together
always. Examples are pectoralis major, gluteus maximus and
the majority of the vertebral muscles.

Every arcuvial muscle is fully stretched by, and only by, a
full swing of the bone(s); it can act on together with a full rotation of the same bone(s) around the shaft (body, *corpus*);
this swing and rotation being, of course, within the limits permitted by the joint(s) involved. Consequently, complete reversal of the said swing and rotation can only be caused by
complete contraction of the muscle with, of course, the reduction or complete undoing of any twist the stretched muscle
may have undergone.

At this point we first define two useful words and then
digress to define and illustrate four necessary words already
long in use, now classical in fact. Then we shall return to
arcuvial muscles.

The "useful" words are *necessarily* and *potentially*, and
refer to the threefold classification of arcuvial muscles that
began this section. Class (i) is necessarily arcuvial. Class (ii)
is potentially arcuvial and potentially chordovial. Class (iii) is
potentially arcuvial, chordovial and gyrovial. We now look at
the "necessary" words.

Prime Movers, Antagonists and Synergists See 205

A muscle is a *prime mover* when it causes at least one of the
actions that it is capable of causing. Thus the brachialis is a
prime mover in flexion of the elbow; but the biceps brachii is
a prime mover in flexion of the elbow, in supination of the
forearm and, of course, in a combination of these two movements.

A muscle is an *antagonist* to a prime mover when it can oppose *all* of the actions of that prime mover. Thus, the
brachialis and triceps brachii are antagonists to each other;
so also are the biceps brachii and the humero-radial supinator — kinematically but not kinetically!

A *synergist* is a muscle that acts with an arcuvial prime
mover as a *partial antagonist* of that prime mover; that is, it
lessens or even prevents at least one of the other two actions
of that muscle. Thus the triceps brachii is a synergist to the
biceps brachii when the biceps supinates but does not flex the
forearm; whereas the pronator quadratus is a synergist to the
biceps when the latter flexes but does not supinate the forearm.

Two muscles are both prime movers and also *co-synergists*
if they both act to produce the same movement of a bone but
act synergically on each other with respect to unwanted
movement(s). Thus the two interossei of a digit are co-
synergists when they both act to produce pure flexion of that
finger on its corresponding metacarpal; here each prevents
the conjunct rotation that its cosynergist would cause. Similarly, the flexor and extensor carpi ulnaris are cosynergists
with respect to ulnar deviation of the hand at the radiocarpal
joint; in this case the flexor action of the first prevents the
extensor action of the second, leaving only the ulnar devia-
tory components of both effective.

The term "synergist" as defined above was first used by
anatomists and in a kinematical sense, and it will be so used
here. It is a Greek form of "collaborator" or fellow-worker.
Later, physiologists (who are fond of Greek) began to use it in
the sense of "co-prime mover"; they use it in a *kinetic* sense;

thus they would class the biceps brachii as a synergist of the brachialis. What they should have done (and should do) is to use the term *synagonist* for what they mean in such cases. We shall do so; for it is the obvious opposite of "antagonist."

Arcuvial Muscles Continued

We can now make clear and relatively brief statements about the myokinematics of arcuvial muscles.

Necessarily arcuvial. These muscles can swing bones only along one path. The amount of conjunct rotation of the bone will increase with the amount of its swing but not exactly proportionally to it.

Potentially chordovial. These muscles can swing bones along a (theoretically infinite) number of paths all of the same sense, clockwise or anticlockwise. The amount of conjunct rotation of the bone will depend upon the particular path, this being determined by the extent to which one or more synergists act upon the bone. When the action of the synergist(s) is complete then the path will be a cardinal (chordal) swing devoid of conjunct rotation.

Potential gyrovial. These muscles are limited to those acting on the radio-humeral, shoulder, hip, and vertebral joints. The first and last groups are simpler to consider than the middle two groups, and will be looked at first.

Pure spin of the radius on the capitulum of the humerus requires a synergic action of an extensor (triceps) when the pronator teres is used; and a flexor synergist is needed if the complete supinator is employed for supination. But the ulnoradial part of the supinator requires no synergist, being gyrovial by itself.

The movements of the backbone were dealt with in the last chapter. Rotation of it is caused by muscles that can also flex or extend it; and also can swing its parts to one side or another. Most of the muscles used for swinging the head and and/or the trunk around the curved long axis of the backbone are cosynergic.

When we come to the femur and humerus we find a clash between the kinematic truth about their motions and the universally accepted naming of them. It was shown in Chapter 3 that the motions of the bodies of these bones are the result of the motions of the parts of the bones called "femorellum" and "humerellus" in the case of femur and humerus, respectively. These parts are wholly intra-articular, and are directed upwards and medially from the shafts. Consequently the motions called flexion and extension of the bones are due to a *spin* of the femurellum and humerellus. But the motions called medial and lateral (inward and outward) rotation of the bones are really forward and backward *swings* of them, respectively; this has recently been demonstrated for the femur radiologically (Hooper and Ormond, 1975).

If, then, we pin our attention on the femur alone, the only potentially gyrovial muscles are those of flexion and extension. But we can and should look further along the limbs.

What we call medial and lateral rotation of the femur and humerus do in fact cause pure spins of the leg and forearm, respectively. When the hip and knee are in extension the "rotations" of the femur cause corresponding true rotations of the leg around a vertical axis passing through the heel, as he easily demonstrated on oneself. Demonstration of the rotations of the forearm are less easy, because they require the forearm to be kept supinated throughout the "rotations" of the humerus. Thus, all of the arcuvial muscles acting on the femur and humerus are also potentially gyrovial with respect to *the limb as a whole;* and, of course, muscles exist to move limbs not only the bones thereof!

The *gyrovial efficiency* of an arcuvial muscle depends upon the position of the bone it acts on. Pure flexion and extension can take place only when the arm or thigh is parallel with the body. In this position the subscapularis passes across the humerus transversely and is then most efficient as a medial rotator of it. As the humerus becomes abducted so does the teres major become more transverse instead of being oblique in its passage around the bone. Finally, the pectoral part of pectoralis major is most transverse, and so most gyrovially efficient, in its circumhumeral course around the laterally rotated bone.

Clinical observation has shown that the total range of rotation of the arm changes from 160° in full abduction to 136° in the vertical position, a drop of 15 per cent. In the case of the femur the change in total range is from 90° in full flexion to 83° in the vertical position, a drop of 8 per cent. These figures have been recorded as averages by the American Academy of Orthopaedic Surgeons (*Joint Motion*, 1965).

Active chordovial insufficiency: The term *active insufficiency* is a very old one; it means the inability of a muscle to move a bone through the whole angle that corresponds to its length and attachments, as this angle would be calculated by one of the three kinematic equations we have given above.

All potentially-chordovial arcuvial muscles are actively insufficient with respect to swing. This is what one would expect without recourse to detailed mathematics. When fully stretched an arcuvial muscle is wrapped around part of the bone on which it exercises its power of spin; and it cannot exercise its full power of pure swing until it has been completely unwrapped. When it has been unwrapped a portion of the muscle's myones will have become non-contractile, for the simple reason that they are already contracted! Thus the muscle has virtually increased the amount of tendon in it; so that the myonemes used for pure swing will have a lesser kinematic *(but not kinetic)* effect than they otherwise would have had. Let us look more closely at this phenomenon.

Consider a fully stretched (arcuvial) myoneme of length s'. A part of this length will be wrapped around the bone. This part will be of length, say, $2aRr$, where a increase from 1 as the myoneme approaches its insertion more and more obliquely; as we have learnt from our study of gyrovial muscles. As the myoneme becomes more and more unwrapped so will $2aRr$ change more and more to aRr. Therefore, the virtual (or effective) length of the myoneme available for pure swing will change from $s' - 2aRr$ to $s' - aRr$. Thus the myonemes involved will become most efficient as chordovial myonemes when they have exercised their power of spin completely. It is enough, therefore, to consider this particular case in detail. The fact that a is unknown to us is of no importance for our purposes.

Let s be the length between the origin of the fully un-wrapped myoneme and the point where it now reaches the bone — its "virtual insertion." The myoneme will cross some axis of swing and we can, therefore, find lengths c and q as in the case of purely chordovial muscles. Hence we can find a partition-ratio p for our now fully "chordovialized" myo-neme — if the reader will permit this term! It might be thought that we could now apply one of the kinematic equa-tions for chordovial muscles immediately, using only p and t as in those equations. This is not so.

The part of s which is aRr is non-contractile and also non-relaxed, so that it is equivalent to tendon. If t be the propor-tion of tendon in the fully stretched myoneme, then the total non-contractile part of s is $(st + aRr)$. The remaining part of s is fully contractile and can, therefore, contract to half its length. The results of these facts are proved in Appendix B; we give them here in brief.

Let F be the actual (angle of) flexion caused by full con-traction of a chordovialized myoneme (and its helpers) and let F' be the flexion that would occur if p and t only were in-volved. Then:

$$sin^2 F/2 = sin^2 F'/2 - ax\ Rr - a^2y^2(Rr)^2$$

where x and y are functions of a, p and t. Similarly, if E and E' be the corresponding extensions caused by myonemes of an extensor muscle we have:

$$sin^2 E/2 = sin^2 E'/2 - axRr + a^2y^2\ (Rr)^2$$

This shows that only if $R = O$ are F and E equal to F' and E', respectively. The interested reader is referred to Appendix B for further details. The quantities a and x differ in the two equations given above.

Since a has its least value ($=1$) when the myonemes are transverse to the bone they act on, it follows that the actual swing and the "ideal" swing will then differ least. That is to say, *for every arcuvial muscle there is an optimal position of the bone,* in which position the muscle produces both its maximal swing and its maximal spin effect *per number of ac-tively contracting myones*. For the biceps brachii this posi-tion is that of right-angled flexion of the elbow. For the ab-ductors of the shoulder it is the position of full abduction or near it, depending on the muscle.

A Note on the Orbital Muscles

Although we are chiefly concerned with skeletal muscles yet the orbital (oculomotor) muscles will be of interest to most readers of this book. All their myonemes are collinear tendonemes, so that we look at these muscles before passing to the pennate kind. Of the four rectus muscles two are chor-dovial, the medial and the lateral; the superior and inferior are arcuvial; so also are the two oblique muscles (fig. 6.9).

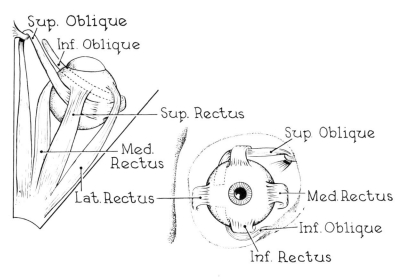

Fig. 6.9. The extra-ocular muscles of the right eye from above and in front.

Most of our muscles are essentially prime movers, though many can be synergic to other muscles as well. *But in each orbit there is a pair of muscles whose function is wholly syn-ergic.* These are the superior and inferior oblique muscles. They are required because of the consequences of diadochal movements of the eyeball.

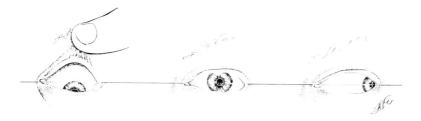

Fig. 6.10. Movements of the left eye as described in the text.

An eye in an orbital cavity is like the head of a femur or humerus in *its* joint cavity, for it is capable of rotating around three principal axes. The cornea can be swung upwards and downwards around a mediolateral axis, medially and later-ally around a vertical axis. In principle it can also be sub-jected to a "spin" around an anteroposterior axis, so that it has 3 potential degrees of freedom of motion. *In normal cases only the swings are allowed, never the spins.* This is be-cause a spin would rotate the retina and literally disorientate it with respect to the field of vision. The subjects would then interpret his retinal picture wrongly; for example, he would see a vertical rod as if it were oblique, as is known from clin-ical ophthalmology for certain kinds of squint (strabismus) in which paralysis of one or other of the two muscles in ques-tion occurs.

Between sleep and sleep, an eye is constantly on the move. It will converge with its fellow upon some near thing, then move upwards and scan some distant view. Movement in one direction follows movement in some other — we have a suc-cession of diadochal swings, just as happens at some joints. Each pair of swings would bring about a conjunct rotation, a spin of the eye, something that we have seen to be unwanted. So we must have synergic, anti-spin muscles. Two are both necessary and sufficient, for a spin can only be clockwise or anticlockwise.

Look at a man's *left* eye (fig. 6.10). He is looking down and then swings his eye up to gaze ahead, at you. He next swings it to the left side. He has thus made a *clockwise* diadochal movement (from your point of view). This entails a potential clockwise spin of his eye, requiring an anticlockwise force-couple (or equivalent) to prevent it. The need is met by the left *superior oblique* muscle, the tendon of which runs across the upper part of the eyeball laterally as well as posteriorly, so that it can exercise the necessary anticlockwise movement upon the eye. Similarly, were the left eye to swing upwards and medially then the *inferior oblique* muscle would exercise the clockwise movement upon the lower part of the eye for preventing the anticlockwise spin that would occur otherwise.

Most men have two eyes which move together rightwards or leftwards in scanning. It follows that when scanning is one part of a diadochal movement then the *superior* oblique of one eye will contract with the *inferior* oblique of the other. Thus a scan to the right following a raising of both eyes will involve (1) the right lateral rectus and superior oblique and (2) the left medial rectus and inferior oblique. But an *immediately* following scan to the left will involve only the left lateral and the right medial recti. In this instance the prime movers require no synergists.

Even when our eyes are in the converged state, as in reading a book, the oblique muscles will come into play, for reading requires movements in both vertical and horizontal directions, hence diadochal movements of the eyes.

Squint is caused by disturbances of the extra-ocular muscles. When these involve one or other of the obliques then retinal spin occurs.

It must be mentioned, however, that *torsion* (spin) of the eyeballs is often required for normal vision. If one's head is bent to the right, a clockwise movement, then both eyes undergo compensatory, anticlockwise spin so that the orientation of the retina relative to the visual field remains constant. This spin is mediated by a complex reflex system involving the vestibular nerves. The amount of such a spin is, however, limited — our eyes do not turn through a right angle when we lay us down to sleep!

Pennate Muscles

A pennate (feather-like) muscle is one whose contractile parts join a common tendon obliquely (fig. 6.11). These parts may join the tendon on one side only *(unipennate)*, on two opposite sides *(bipennate)* or from all sides *(circumpenate)*.

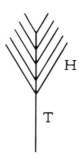

Fig. 6.11. Diagram of part of a bipennate muscle. H: holonemic part. T: part of the tendon.

Visibly pennate muscles are found in the limbs; they act on joints other than the hip and shoulder. The middle part of the deltoid muscle, which acts on the shoulder, consists of a number of pennate muscles; the upper set acts on the tendons of the lower set, and it is these tendons which pull on the humerus. This muscle is therefore called *multipennate*.

Every pennate muscle passes over at least two joints. One of these is its *principal joint*, that to which its main action is directed. Thus the tendon of flexor hallucis longus (unipennate) passes over the radiocarpal, lateral carpal, and all of the thumb's joints, but its main action is on the interphalangeal joint of the thumb.

Spin d swing

Every pennate muscle is arcuvial. Excepting the interossei, its main action brings its principal joint *out of* the close-packed position by an arcuate swing. The interossei, however, are potentially chordovial. They bring the MP joints *into* the close-packed position, *either* by acting together co-synergically and chordovially *or* by acting in sequence to produce arcuate motions of opposite sense successively.

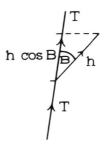

Fig. 6.12. The action of the contractile part of a pennate myoneme upon its tendinous part. See text.

We now define and consider the action of a *pennate myoneme.* It consists of two parts (fig. 6.12):

i) *The contractile part:* this is a holoneme making an angle B with the common tendon.

ii) *The tendinous part:* this is all that part of the common tendon that runs from the attachment of the contractile part to the attachment of the tendon on the mobile bone of the muscle's principal joint. Thus the tendinous parts of pennate myonemes become shorter as their points of attachment progress further along the common tendon. But t, the proportion of tendon in the whole myoneme, is always very large — from 70 to 90 per cent.

In a fully stretched myoneme the angle B has a range of 0 to 30°. For the uppermost part of the muscle the range of B is from 0 to 10°, so that the myonemes here are actually or virtually collinear.

The simplest way to describe the action of a pennate myoneme or muscle is to say that it is kinematically less efficient
than the collinear type — in the ancient engineer's sense; for
he would measure its efficiency by the angle of swing and/or
rotation per unit of energy used. But the body's standards of
efficiency are not necessarily those of the ancient engineer, a
fact to be remembered by those who propose to become bio-
engineers.

The reason for the diminished efficiency is shown in fig.
6.12. Let the holonemic (contractile) part of a pennate myoneme have a length h when fully stretched. Then the system
is *as if* the myonemes were collinear with an initial length h
cos B. Simple trigonometry shows that when h contracts to
$h/2$ then the tendon will be pulled through a distance less
than $h/2$. If this distance be d, then the actual equation is

$$d = (s\text{-}z) = \frac{h}{2}\left(2 - \sqrt{1 - sin^2 B}\right)$$

The full theory of pennate muscles will be found in Mac-
Conaill (1971). Here we give two examples of the diminished
kinematic efficiency of the pennate type. We first note, however, that if a pennate myoneme were one unit long and B
were 30 per cent, then it would be equivalent to a collinear
holoneme of 0.886 unit long; that is, the efficiency of its
linear pull would be reduced to under 90 per cent. This is a
useful standard or a "yardstick."

The *flexor pollicis longus* flexes the terminal phalanx of the
thumb (when the muscle is fully stretched to begin with)
through 90°. In a typical instance we find, using symbols now
familiar to the reader: $s = c\text{+}q = 30$ cm; $q = 0.5$ cm; $st = 28$ cm.
From these data we obtain $p = 59$ and $t = 14/15$. Applying
these values of p and t to the kinematic equation for collinear
chordovial muscles, we find that a non-pennate muscle
would flex the phalanx through 128°. Hence the efficiency of
the actual muscle is 90/128, that is, 70 per cent in units of
swing.

Our second example is the *rectus femoris*, a muscle easily
studied in living subjects. It extends the knee through a total

range of 144°. Its muscular part extends almost the whole length of the thigh. The terminal part of its tendon is the *quadriceps femoris* tendon, which includes the patella and the so-called ligamentum patellae, by which the muscle is inserted into uppermost part of the front of the tibia. It can be mapped easily in living subjects and its fully stretched length (*s*) and fully contracted length found by using a flexible measuring tape.

The rectus femoris is a "pulley-muscle" (*musculus trochlearis*) and acts by pulling the tibia forwards around the curved articular surfaces of the two femoral condyles (when the leg and foot are mobile). These condyles are spiral in outline; but when we are dealing with the *total* amount of flexion we can take them to be equivalent to circles, each having a radius which has the average value of the radius of curvature of the spin at successive points. Thus we can apply the formula for *gyrovial* muscles in this instance without serious error; and equate the shortening in length of the muscle with Rr, where R is total angle of extension (in radians) and r is the said average radius of curvature of the muscle insertion. The said shortening in length is, of course, that which should occur if the muscle were collinear.

In a typical instance the following data were found: $s = 52$ cm; $z = 44$ cm; $r = 3$ cm; $s\text{-}z = 8$ cm. Since 144° is 2.5 radians, the shortening for a collinear type of rectus femoris would be Rr, that is 7.5 cm. The efficiency of the actual muscle is, therefore, 75/80, that is, 93.6 per cent. This figure is for extension of the knee with the hip in extension. The high efficiency of the muscle, measured in terms of *actual* compared with *ideal* shortening, is probably correlated with the fact that it is also a flexor of the hip — it is a *biarticular muscle*. This brings us to a brief consideration of multi-articular muscles.

Multiarticular Muscles

A muscle that can act on two or more joints in series is called *multiarticular*. Some multiarticular muscles always

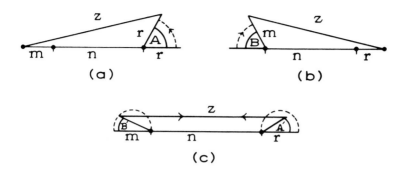

Fig. 6.13. Diagram of a biarticular myoneme. For details see text.

act on all the joints they pass over, others do not. Thus the flexores and extensores carpi act on all the joints they pass over; but the rectus femoris can act on the knee alone, on the hip alone or on both joints at the same time.

According to the number of joints they act on, so are these muscles classified as biarticular, triarticular, and so on. They can also be classified as *linear* or *spiral*: the classification refers to the fully contracted muscle. A linear muscle remains on the same side of the trunk or limb from origin to insertion; a spiral muscle does not. Thus the rectus femoris is linear but the sartorius is spiral.

The possible actions of a multiarticular muscle follow from the fact that the muscle contracts as a whole whether it be acting on one or more joints — it has not separately contractile parts for each joint; together with the laws of approximation and detorsion. *Three useful rules*, easily verified by the reader, can be stated:

i) The *swings* at the joints acted on by a linear muscle are all of the same sense; but are of opposite sense if the muscle be spiral.

ii) The *spins* at the joints acted on by either a linear or a spiral muscle are *all of the same sense*, whether the muscle be linear or spiral. In a word, they are *congruent* (Chapter 5).

iii) The *amount* of swing and/or spin produced by the muscle is always greatest at any joint when only that joint is permitted to move.

Rule (i) follows from the law of approximation: a muscle brings its bones of origin and of insertion nearer to each other if both are free to move. Thus rectus femoris brings hipbone and tibia nearer to the femur by flexing the first and extending the second by swings of the same sense. But the sartorius, passing from front to back of femur swings the hipbone and tibia nearer to the femur by motions of opposite senses.

Rule (ii) follows from the law of detorsion. If the spins of any two bones moved by one and the same muscle were in opposite directions then the contracting muscle would become more, instead of less, twisted; and this is contrary to the said law.

Rule (iii) is a matter of simple geometry. It is best explained by considering a biarticular myoneme, as shown in fig. 6.13. This itself represents a simple model that the reader could easily make.

The figure shows a myoneme (or bundle of parallel myonemes) that can act on each of two bones articulating with an intermediate bone of length n. The myoneme is attached to one bone at a distance m from its axis of swing, and to the other at a distance r from this other's axis of swing. The myoneme is obviously linear. For clarity, let the first of the bones (left-hand side in the figure) be called the initial bone, and the second (most right-hand in the figure) be called the terminal bone. And for simplicity let the myoneme have its fully stretched length (s) when both joints are in extension, as shown.

First let only the terminal bone be mobile, and let the myoneme contract to its minimal length z. Then the terminal bone will swing through an angle A. If the myoneme be chordovial, then A will be determined by the proportion of tendon t and by a p here equal to $(m+n)/r$; and A is the maximal swing of the terminal bone (fig. 6.13 a). Next, let the initial bone be the mobile one. In this case contraction s to z will swing it through an angle B (fig. 13 b); now p will be $(n+r)/m$; and A and B will be equal if and only if $m = r$, since s, t and z are the same in both cases.

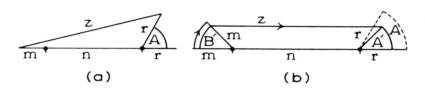

Fig. 6.14. To illustrate the concept of active insufficiency of muscle. Details in text. The arrow in b shows the direction in which z is "moved" because of the permitted mobility of m. A: maximal value of swing of r: A': reduced swing because of motion of m.

Finally let both the initial and terminal bones be mobile. The extremities of both m and r will move in curved paths; there is no loss of generality in assuming that the two paths are arcs of circles, as in fig. 6.14. Diagram (a) in this figure is a repetition of diagram (a) in the previous figure; diagram (b) shows both bones mobile and swung through angles A' and B' instead of A and B, respectively. Because m, n, r and z are unchanged in length, the only possible change is in the position of z. As the extremity of m moves through B' so must that of r move along its arc in *the same sense* as that of m; hence A' will be less than A. By similar reasoning B' is less than B.

Hence if both bones be mobile the muscle cannot move at least one of them through its fullest angle of swing. The same can be proved easily for angles of spin. This is another example of active insufficiency of a muscle.

The biarticular type is well represented by the long flexors of the knee, which are also extensors of the hip; these are the biceps femoris (long head), the semitendinosus and the semimembranosus. The rectus femoris is another good example; it is a flexor of the hip and extensor of the knee.

The multiarticular type is well represented by the long muscles of the vertebral column.

When a bi- or multiarticular muscle moves all the bones it can act upon then the actual motion of each bone (therefore the degree of active insufficiency of the muscle) will depend upon *kinetic* factors. Further, for z in fig. 6.14 we could substitute z', a lesser length than z, and the geometrical demonstration of active insufficiency would still be valid.

Value of the Kinematic Equations

The kinematic equations for chordovial and gyrovial muscles (given on pages 104 and 111) may seem useless theory, since the vast majority of muscles are arcuvial. But, as our study of biarticular muscles has shown, these equations provide a meaningful standard by which to assess the "efficiency" of a muscle in terms of its actual performance compared with a theoretical value based on the functional essentials of its structure — its partition-ratio, its tendon-proportion, and its amount of winding around the bone it acts on.

The General Rule of Myokinematics

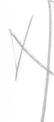

Finally, we give a general rule for determining the possible kinematic actions of any skeletal muscle: if any normal movement of a bone would stretch and/or twist a muscle, then the possible kinematic actions of that muscle will be those which would reduce that stretching and/or twisting. This rule can be applied by any person looking at a dissection of the part of the body involved and using his or her imagination. In applying the rule the effect of a conjunct rotation in stretching or twisting the muscle should always be remembered.

REFERENCES

Hooper, A.C. and Ormond, D.J. (1975) A radiographic study of hip rotation. *Ir. J. Med. Sc., 144:* 25-29.

MacConaill, M.A. (1971) The kinematic anatomy of skeletal muscle fibres. 1: Basic principles. *Ir. J. Med. Sc., 140:* 387-402.

MacConaill, M.A. (1973) The psalloscope and its uses. *Lo Scalpello,* pp. 285-290.

Sissons, H.A. (1969) Anatomy of the motor unit. In: *Disorders of Voluntary Muscle,* pp. 1-16. Churchill, London.

SEVEN

The Potential Actions of Muscles: Kinetic

Muscles cannot exercise their kinematic powers unless they have the necessary and sufficient forces to move or stabilize the parts on which they act. The study of these forces is called Myokinetics.

Myokinetics is divisible into two parts, myostatics and myo-dynamics; the first deals with the stabilization of bones (and their loads) in some position or other, the second deals with their movements into or out of these positions. Myostatics is actually a limiting (or special) case of myodynamics, that in which the speed of movement is *nil;* and a most important problem in it cannot be solved until we come to myodynamics. But, as in schoolday physics, it is better to study the static (or stabilizing) use of muscles first.

Unless we are among the few who roam in outer space, gravity is always with us. Our muscles are designed or evolved (or both) to act against it, be it for stabilization or for movement. Every muscle is an anti-gravitational muscles in some position or another. So the greater part of our study will take full account of gravity as the force against which our muscles act, at least when we are "up and about." In plain words, we shall remember that every part of a body has a weight against which myokinetic forces not only act but can be measured.

"*Bones.*" The word *bone* will mean not only the actual bone on which a muscle acts but also the total load that is stabilized or moved when the bone itself is stabilized or moved; unless we are talking of the bone itself, when this fact will be stated clearly. Thus *ulna* will mean not only this anatomical structure

131

but also the forearm together with the hand and fingers and any additional load carried by any of these parts.

This definition of "bone" will not be repeated. The word is short, and its definition makes it exact. Of course, anyone who wishes to substitute "osseo-musculo-vasculo-cutaneous mass" for it is at liberty to do so!

Plan of this Chapter

The purpose of this part of the book is to show how the structure and arrangement of skeletal muscles is related to their ability to perform various tasks, all of which require the expenditure of energy. It begins with a look at the four possible states of living myonemes (and hence of muscles); passes to the basic kinetics of myonemes; then to myostatics; then to myodynamics; and finally to the statement of certain tentative laws of muscle action with the limitations imposed by bodily structure upon their invariable operation.

When we come to myodynamics we take note of the fact that all muscle action is completely controlled, both in amount and in speed, by the central nervous system. This fact appears to be ignored often by would-be biomechanicians, who seem to think of the locomotor system as a kind of automobile engine governed by schoolbook physics. It is certainly mobile but it is not *auto*-mobile.

We shall have to construct and use mathematical equations and also "inequalities," just as in kinematics. Space does not allow of these equations being arrived at step by step. So the non-mathematical reader is asked either to accept them, or, better, to ask a mathematical friend to verify them from the data. Numerical examples are given where they are relevant. To assist reference to earlier equations every equation of importance is numbered; by "of importance" is meant that it is in its final form should it depend upon some equation preceding it.

Symbols. All undefined symbols used will have the meanings given to them in myokinematics. Thus c, q and p (= c/q)

will mean what they did in Chapter 6. Other symbols will be defined as need arises.

Only two Greek letters are used. One is ρ (to be defined later). The other is π, the usual mathematical symbol for the number 3.14. . .; thus π radians = 180°. We would recall that such an expression as $cosA/2$ is to be read as $cos(A/2)$ — this is for convenience in printing, and will in fact cause no confusion.

The Four States of Living Muscle

A myoneme may be in any one of four states at any given time. These states are:

i) Relaxed without change of length (isometric relaxation);

ii) Relaxed and stretched (anisometric relaxation);

iii) Hardened (isometric contraction); and

iv) Shortened and hardened (isotonic contraction).

The first two terms explain themselves. So also do the second two; but the names for them in parentheses are names given to them by 19th century physiologists and still used by their 20th century successors. The first of these names is absurd; if something contracts it cannot retain its length (isometric). The second is wrong: muscle fibres (cells or myonemes) have their greatest strength (*tonus*) when they are fully stretched — so they cannot preserve that strength (be isotonic) as they shorten. We shall use the familiar and accurate terms (MacConaill, 1973), except that *contraction* will denote 'shortening and hardening.'

Hardened and, of course, shortened muscles exert *active forces*. Relaxed, and even more, stretched muscles exert *reactive forces*; for energy is required to stretch them and they oppose a *visco-elastic resistance* to stretching: this resistance is now taken note of by all myologists.

An active force is so called because it is caused by energy generated within the muscle; even hardening requires the use of muscle energy. A reactive force is so called because the energy causing it is supplied from some source external to the muscle. If this energy be applied either too suddenly or in too great measure, the muscle may break, completely or incompletely.

That a muscle hardens when it contracts and that it can harden without shortening are both easily demonstrated upon the reader's first dorsal interosseus muscles by means of a finger of the other hand applied to that on which the muscle to be tested is. The combined swelling and hardening of the contracting muscle are very easily felt; the hardening of the muscle when either radial deviation of the index or flexion of it at the metacarpo-phalangeal joint are resisted is also appreciable by a finger pushed against the skin of the region between the first and second metacarpals. This is, of course, a special case of the technique of "resisted contraction" used by many, possibly by all, readers for making muscles palpable.

The First Purpose of Myokinetics

The first purpose of myokinetics is to determine the *total* force that is *both necessary and sufficient* for either the stabilization of a bone or for moving it at some chosen rate of speed without the danger of dislocation of the joint at which the bone is stabilized or moved. "Dislocation" does not mean only the kind of accident that calls for surgical treatment. It includes any loss of contact between a resting bone and its conarticular bone at the articular unit involved. It also includes any separation of a moving bone and its conarticular fellow other than by the very thin film of synovial fluid that is necessary for lubrication; this film is exceedingly thin and is measured in micro-millimetres.

Except in the close-packed position, the capsule and ligaments of a joint are quite unable to prevent dislocation as it has just been defined. What does prevent it is a force acting along the fixed or moving bone, the transarticular force, which is generated by muscles and/or gravity. It will be shown that it is a constant in all positions of a fixed bone of constant load; and it is increased during a swing by the centripetal force that invariably accompanies that swing and which is proportional to the load (weight) of the moving bone.

The primary function of muscles is to cause movement. This is not an empty statement. When muscles assist in stabilizing a bone they act as rather expensive ligaments — expensive in the sense that they use energy in doing so. We should not be surprised, therefore, at finding such quantities as the transarticular force determined by the *principle of muscular economy* as it operates in myodynamics, not as some would think it should operate in myostatics. It does in fact operate in myostatics insofar as the "resting" positions of the head, trunk and limbs of a standing (or sitting) person are those in which gravity is the principal force for stabilization of those parts. And, of course, when we lie upon a bed, couch, table or the ground, muscular force is used minimally — if we know how to relax!

Finally, it must be stressed that not everyone uses minimal muscular force for moving bones. The art of doing so has to be learnt from infancy onwards by "trial and error." Those who correct the errors we call "skilled," those who do not we call "clumsy." This is a point that should always be kept in mind when the results of EMG experiments made on random samples of individuals are compared with myokinetic theory of the kind to be developed here.

The Forces Exerted by Muscles

Let a muscle act upon a bone — an actual bone this time, either by simple hardening or by contracting. Then it will pull on the bone with a certain force F directed along its own length (fig. 7.1). This force is resolvable (in the general case) into three component forces, all acting on the bone's surface. These components are: a *swing force* (A), a *spin force* (rotational force) R, and a transarticular muscle-force T.

We can thus write an equation:

(1) $F = T + A + R$

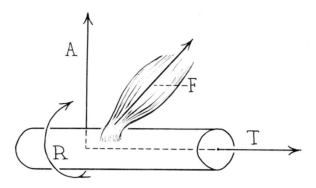

Fig. 7.1. The three major components into which the force (F) of a muscle acting upon a bone is resolved. A, force across the long axis of the bone; R, the rotational (spin) component; T, the transarticular component, the arrow pointing towards the joint.

This is a vector equation, for each of its parts has not only an amount (magnitude) but also a sense (direction) and is therefore called a *vector*. If vector algebra were understood outside the world of professional physicists and engineers, this chapter could be compressed into a few pages. Unless vectors are (a) all of the same kind (forces, speeds, etc.) and (b) parallel to one another, they cannot be added or subtracted by simple arithmetic. Quantities that can be added and subtracted in that way are called *scalars*.

Nevertheless, equation (1) is useful. It represents the complete action of an arcuial muscle. One component (A) is chordoval; a second (R) is gyroval; the third (T) is potentially kinematic, for it could move the bone along its own axis if it were not resisted by the articular surface of the bone's conarticular partner. We shall study A and T together, leaving R until later.

Note: from now onwards the symbols A, R and T will have different meanings from those given to them above — TAR is only a useful aid to memory.

The Kinetics of a Swing Myoneme

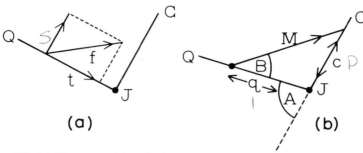

Fig. 7.2. (a) The spurt (s) and shunt (t) components of a force f acting on a bone Q. (b) A myoneme M extends from Q to its conarticular bone C. The arrows show the direction of action of forces (see text). J is the position of the swing-axis of the joint between C and Q.

Every active myoneme is a visible "line of force," a visible vector, for the force it produces acts along it in the direction of its pull. Thus the kinetics of a myoneme is that of the force it produces at any instant.

A myoneme can be represented by a line in a diagram. So also can a bone if we are studying swings alone. Hence we can draw the diagram shown in fig. 7.2.

In (a) of fig. 7.2 we see two bones C and Q, one of which swings upon the other around an axis at J. This axis is perpendicular to both C and Q (and to the page). Q has been already swung through an angle A out of full collinearity (extension) with C, its original position being shown by the broken line Q'.

A force of amount f acts on some point of Q in the direction of C. This force is generated by a myoneme (not shown) that makes an angle B with Q; this angle is always measured on the side of a myoneme nearer to C (or J). The force has two components: a swing-force at right angles to Q, and a transarticular force along Q. Whatever geometrical theory may permit, *the transarticular component of myonemic force always presses the affected bone towards the articular surface of the conarticular bone.* This is true whether the myoneme be flexor or extensor, abductor or adductor.

We denote the swing force by s and the transarticular force by t, these letters being no longer required (for the present) in their kinematic sense. It appears from elementary mechanics that:

$$(2) \quad s = f \sin B; \quad t = f \cos B$$

Thus if f were 5 units (lb. or million-dynes) and B were 37°, then s would be 3 units and t would be 4 units; for 3/5 and 4/5 are $\sin 37°$ and $\cos 37°$, respectively. But if B were 53° then s would be 4 units and t would be 3 units, for $\sin 53°$ and $\cos 53°$ are 4/5 and 3/5 respectively. In both cases B has been given to the nearest degree for the sines and cosines used as illustrations.

Spurt and Shunt Forces. The components s and t could be called "transaxial" and "paraxial" forces, since they act directly across and directly along the long axis of the bone, respectively. These names were introduced into kinesiology by MacConaill (1946), to replace the misleading terms "phasic" forces and "postural" forces, respectively. A phasic force was so called because it changed the position of a bone, a postural force was supposed to maintain the position of a bone. In fact both functions can be carried out by spurt forces in all circumstances unless when a person is lying on some horizontal structure.

The aforesaid engineers were interested in moving structures. They saw shunt forces as keeping, say, the hub of a wheel pressed against the curved axle on which the wheel turned; and thought of these forces as "shunting" each part of the wheel along the curved line of motion. "Shunt" was really a short word for "centripetal." To use the terms 'spurt force' and 'shunt force' in the senses defined above is like using 'swing' for "motion of a bone around an axis normal to its conarticular surface at an articular unit."

As we prefer brevity to unhelpful prolixity, we shall continue to use all these four words as they have been defined already.

The Spurt-Ratio. The term *spurt-ratio* is short for "spurt-shunt-ratio," that is, the ratio of the spurt to the shunt force of a myoneme (or muscle). Denoting it by S, we have, from equation 2:

$$(3) \quad S = s/t = \tan B$$

In (b) of fig. 7.2 we see the same bones as before, A being unchanged. A myoneme M is attached to C at a distance c from J, and to Q at a distance q from J. Thus M has a partition-ratio p, which is c/q. By elementary geometry we can find that:

$$(4) \quad S = tan\ B = \frac{p\ sin\ A}{1 + p\ cos\ A}$$

Thus the spurt-ratio is expressible wholly in terms of p and A at any instant.

This equation can be given a simple numerical meaning. The greatest possible value of A is 143° (to within one degree); the sine and cosine of this angle are 3/5 and -4/5, respectively. Hence as A passes from 0° through 90° to 143° so does S pass from 0 through p to $3p/(5-4p)$.

It will be shown later that as A increases from 90° to 143° so does p decrease to 1. Hence S is always positive. This means that the shunt force is always positive, for the spurt force is never negative. And this in turn means that *all myonemes generate transarticular forces directed towards, not away from, the joints at which they act.* This law must, therefore, be true for muscles also, for these are simply bundles of myonemes.

When A = 143° (elbow, knee) and p = 1 we have S = 3; that is, spurt force = 3 times shunt force. When A = 90° S = p, so that if $p > 1$ then the shunt force is greater than the spurt. What do these figures mean biologically?

Motor versus Safety Forces. Reference to fig. 7.2 will show that only s can help to move (or stabilize) a bone and only t can contribute to the safety of the joint; that is, prevent it from being dislocated. We can therefore call s the *motor* force and t the *safety* force, so that the ratio S is the ratio of the motor to the safety components of the total force f.

Reference to equation (4) will show that when B = 45° and $tan\ B$ = 1 then we must have

$$(5) \quad sinA - cosA = 1/p$$

This equation means that only if $p > 1$ can $tan\ B$ = 45°. For if $p < 1$ then $1/p$ must be n where $n > 1$. Now ($sinA - cosA$) can never be greater than 1; and this proves the theorem.

It follows that we can divide myonemes sharply into 2 classes: those in which $p \geqslant 1$ and those in which $p < 1$. These two classes are biomechanically distinct. Myonemes for which $p \geqslant 1$ always have the spurt-ratio less than one: in them the safety (shunt) component is always greater than the motor (spurt) component. Myonemes for which $p \gg 1$ always have the motor component greater than the safety component after $(sinA - cosA) > 1/p$; but this cannot occur until $A > 45°$.

Spurt and Shunt Myonemes. On the basis of equations (4) and (5) then, we shall classify myonemes into two types: spurt myonemes and shunt myonemes. The classification is determined by the partition-ration p, which has already been seen to be a basic factor in myokinematics. In the spurt class are all those for which $p \geqslant 1$; the remainder being of the shunt type.

This classification is not due to our excessive love of the terms 'spurt' and 'shunt.' We cannot use the words 'motor' and 'safety' as a basis of classification, because both types of myonemes have motor powers. Neither is the classification invalid because spurt myonemes do not exhibit their "spurtness" until $A > 45°$. To say it is invalid for this reason would be like saying that a child is not to be called human until it has reached a certain stage in its postnatal development.

Loci of Myoneme Types. We have seen that the functional classification of myoneme types (with respect to myokinetics) can be made on a purely anatomical basis. Examination of human muscles shows that:

    i) All extensor and adductor myonemes are of the spurt type; and

    ii) Flexor and abductor myonemes can be of either type.

Reversal of Myoneme Type. Spurt and shunt myonemes are classified as such by reference to their origins and insertions as given in anatomical textbooks. If, however, the direction of a myoneme's pull be reversed then a spurt myoneme becomes a shunt myoneme and a shunt myoneme becomes a spurt myoneme; unless, of course, $p = 1$ (which is uncommon).

This is because a partition-ratio p becomes $1/p$ if the direction of pull be reversed. Such a reversal makes no difference to the *kinematic* effect and properties of the myoneme, but it does make a difference to its *kinetic* properties.

Hence a knowledge of the anatomical origins of myonemes (and muscles) with respect to the axes of movement produced by them is far from being that "useless information" which it is proclaimed to be by those "up-to-date" slashers of anatomical teaching who want us to go back to a mediaeval knowledge of the structure of the body. Fortunately, they are confined mainly to the Anglo-Saxon cultural sphere.

Limits to Myonemic Force. When $B = 90°$ then *tan B* is infinity; this means that the shunt force is 0 and that all the force of the myoneme would be then of the motor (spurt) kind. There is, however, another possibility, namely, that the myoneme goes out of action so that $f = 0$. If this did not happen, then any further increase of B would not only reduce the amount of the spurt force but also make the shunt force negative; that is, it would act to pull (or help to pull) the bone away from the joint and therefore be an anti-safety force. Biomechanically this would be a bad thing. When we come to consider myostatics it will be shown that the available experimental evidence is in favour of the rule that the myonemes do go out of action when $B = 90°$.

Equivalent Myonemes

So far we have been looking at single myonemes; this was sufficient for our purposes. But a single myoneme is useless by itself; stabilization and motion are caused by those bundles of myonemes that are contained in the named muscles of the body. For the present we are not concerned with these muscles as such, but only with the total forces they exert. For this purpose we consider the total muscular force at any instant (i.e. for any angle A) to be generated by what we call an *equivalent myoneme.*

Look again at fig. 7.1b. If we now think of the myoneme M shown in it as a "super-powerful" myoneme, for which f is now the *total* force exerted by a muscle or a set of muscles, then M is an equivalent myoneme.

The concept of equivalent myonemes has in fact been used *implicitly* for some 300 years; for the representation of a total muscular force by a single line has been used over all that period, long before the word "myoneme" was invented. We have made this concept explicit because it enables us to use the partition-ratio in myokinetics as well as in myokinematics; this is because for every myoneme, including the equivalent type, there is a definite p.

We shall make abundant use of this concept from now onwards.

The Moment of a Force

The word *force* is familiar to all but the term "moment of a force," usually contracted to *moment*, is perhaps not quite so familiar. But it is of primary importance that it should be well understood. This is because the motor effect of a force is dependent upon the moment it exerts upon a bone, whereas the safety effect depends only upon the transarticular (shunt) component of the force itself.

We first define the term "moment" and then state what it means. The definition will be found in all textbooks of physics; the meaning will not!

Definition of Moment. Let any force of amount f act on a bone at a distance q from the axis of swing and make an angle B with the long axis of the bone (Fig. 7.2). Let M then be the magnitude of the moment of force. Then:

$$(6) \quad M = fq \sin B$$

$$(6.1) \quad M = \text{spurt force} \times \text{its distance from axis of swing.}$$

The technical name for the moment is "the moment of the force about the axis of swing;" but the simple term "moment" is sufficient for use since no other axis is involved.

The Meaning of 'Moment.' A moment of force is a *vector*, like the force itself. Its magnitude is that defined above and its direction is that of the spurt force causing it. It could be described as a "directed energy" or as "vectorial energy" whose magnitude can vary from 0 (when $B = 0$) to fq (when

$B = 90°$). A shorter name for it would be "spurt energy."*

This way of thinking about moments may help to make clearer what part they play in myomechanics. We now define a term and then consider equal and unequal moments.

Postaxial Distance. If a force acts on a bone at a distance q from the axis of swing then q will be called the *postaxial distance* (of the point of application of the force). Thus the amount of the corresponding moment is the product of the spurt force by its postaxial distance.

Equal Moments. Let the strength (amount), postaxial distance and angle of pull of one force be f, q, and B, respectively; and let the corresponding parameters ("measures") of a second force be f', q', and B'. Then the moments M and M' of the two forces will be equal if and only if $f' q' sinB' = fq sinB$; that is, if:

$$(7) \quad f' sinB' = f(q/q') sinB$$

If two moments are equal in amount but opposite in direction then the total moment acting on the bone is $(M - M')$, that is, 0.

Unequal Moments. If two moments, M and M', act on the same side of a bone the total moment acting on it is $(M + M')$. But if the two moments act on opposite sides of the bone then the total moment acting on it will be $(M - M')$; and if M and M' are unequal motion will occur.

We are now in a position to study gravitational kinetics and then to study myokinetics in the light of it.

Gravitational Kinetics

Gravitational force is a long name for weight. We shall use

---

*To describe a moment as a directed or vectorial energy may shock some physicists. But, using their special jargon, the 'Dimensions' of a moment are those of energy, that is $[ML^2 T^{-2}]$; and it is absurd not to take note of the fact, even although 'energy' called simply by that name is a scalar quantity. Moreover, parallel and antiparallel moments can be added and subtracted just like scalars, an additional reason for describing (*not* defining) them as energies. After all, physicists now attribute "charm" to certain nuclear entities!

the shorter name as much as possible.

The Gravicentre. Physics permits us to consider the whole weight of a bone (in its general sense) to be concentrated at a single point in the actual bone. We shall call this point the *gravicentre* (G in fig. 7.3). This is a single word for "centre of gravity."

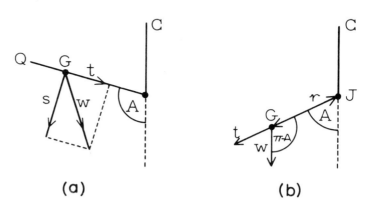

(a)   **(b)**

Fig. 7.3. The spurt (*s*) and shunt (*t*) components of the weight (*w*) of a bone Q. G, gravicentre of Q. Observe the difference between the direction of *t* in (a) and in (b). Further details in text.

The stabilization or movement of a bone thus becomes the fixation or the movement of the gravicentre, as the case may be.

The Graviradius. The postaxial distance of a gravicentre will be called the *graviradius.* It will always be denoted by *r* (fig. 7.3).

The length of *r* has a certain primary value for each bone; this is about half the length of the bone when it is unloaded externally. Thus it is about half the length of a phalanx of a finger; but about half the length from elbow joint to the head of the 3rd phalanx in a postcubitum (forearm + hand). It lengthens if an external weight be borne near or at the termination of the bone; thus it would be at or even beyond the radiocarpal joint if a heavy load were carried by the hand.

We shall, of course, be mostly concerned with the primary length of r.

The Gravitational Force. The weight of a bone is a vector of constant direction (always towards the ground) passing vertically through the gravicentre. If this weight remains constant in any given instance of motion or stability then the vector is a constant vector in the physical sense. Weight will always be denoted by w.

Gravitational Spurt and Shunt. Weight can be also resolved into a spurt and a shunt force (fig. 7.3). If a bone has been swung through an angle A from a vertical line below its joint then the force we are studying makes an angle $(\pi - A)$ with the bone $(\pi + 180°)$. Then geometry assures us that:

(8)   Gravitational spurt force = $w \sin A$

Gravitational shunt force = $-w \cos A$

Before considering the kinesiological significance of these equations we must define two terms of position.

Pendency and antipendency. There are two possible extreme positions of a bone, of any bone. They are defined with respect to gravity but, of course, they can then be used in other contexts. These positions are the pendent and the antipendent.

The *pendent position* is that in which the force of gravity acts along a bone's long axis *and also tends to separate it from its conarticular bone;* that is, to dislocate the joint by direct traction.

The *antipendent position* is that in which the force of gravity acts along the bone's long axis *and also presses the two conarticular surfaces of the relevant articular unit together.* This definition assumes that the lower conarticular surface faces the upper more or less directly; and this is always the case in practice.

Examples of the two positions for the chief bones (or sets of bones) of a standing man are given in fig. 7.4. In this figure the right upper limb is pendent at all joints, the left is antipendent. The curvatures of the backbone prevent all but a few of its vertebrae being precisely antipendent, but the vertebral

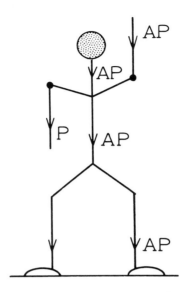

Fig. 7.4. Diagrammatic mannikin to illustrate the concepts of the pendent (P) and antipendent (AP) position of bones.

column *as a whole* is antipendent in a standing or sitting person. In the case of the backbone the joints affected are the intervertebral discs, not the synovial joints.

If a standing man raises one lower limb off the ground then the limb becomes pendent and its muscles now act from above, not from below (if they do act).

Variation of Gravitational Forces. As a bone is swung from the pendent to the antipendent position so does A increase from 0° to 180° (π). This leads to variations of both spurt and shunt forces in accordance with Eqn. (8). It should be noted that although a bone can never swing through 180° at its own joint, yet it can be made antipendent by a movement of its con-articular bone at a joint nearer to the midline of the body; see next section (on Work).

The spurt force of gravity changes from 0 to w and back to 0 as A changes from 0 to 90° to 180°.

The shunt force of gravity changes steadily from -w to 0 and then to w during the same sequence of changes of A.

It is clear that the range of major effect of the spurt force of gravity is in the interval between $A = 45°$ and $A = 135°$.

On the other hand, the shunt force is an *anti-safety* force (in decreasing measure) as A changes from 0 to 90°; and a *safety force* (in increasing measure) as A passes from 90° to 180°. From this latter fact it follows that the *minimal shunt force* operative upon an antipendent bone is w; for if it were less then the bone would be dislocated vertically upwards by gravity! It follows further that no muscular force is *necessary* to stabilize an antipendent bone, its own weight being sufficient for this purpose (so far as swing is involved). This has been verified by EMG; for example, by Joseph and Nightingale (1956) for the hip-joint. Other examples will be found in the chapters dealing with muscles.

Again, if a pendent bone be in its close-packed position at a joint then no force other than that necessary for maintaining that position should be needed. This has been verified by Travill (1962) for the forearm bones; in this case the ulna is maintained in close-pack with the humerus by the anconeus muscle and so needs no antigravitational muscles.

Actually an antipendent bone is not made stable but *metastable* by its weight. It can be disturbed by motions elsewhere in the body and is then brought back to metastability by muscular action (see Part 3).

The Moment of Weight. For clarity, the moment of weight will be denoted by W. We have then:

$$(9) \quad W = wr \, sinA$$

If w be constant, so also will r be, and W will vary exactly as $sin\,A$ does. But if w be increased by a terminal load, r will also increase, so that the moment will increase by an amount greater than w.

Work Against Gravity

All muscular action, be it for stabilization of a bone or for moving it; all such action (we say) involves the expenditure of energy. When that expenditure produces motion of a bone we follow the custom of our engineers and say that *work* is done upon the bone *by* the muscles involved; and we measure the energy expended by measuring the work done. How?

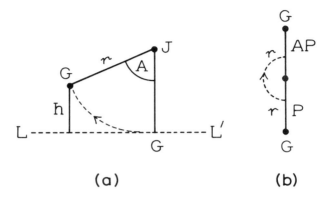

(a)   **(b)**

Fig. 7.5. To illustrate the concept of the work done when a gravicentre (G) is swung through an angle A from pendency at a joint J; *r*, postaxial distance of G; LL′, initial level of G; *h*, vertical displacement of G from LL′.

Let the gravicentre of a bone move from the pendent position to some other by means of a swing of $A°$. In doing so it will move along a curved path. But it will also be displaced *in effect* from its lowest possible position along a *vertical straight line* of height h, as shown in fig. 7.5. This line passes through the gravicentre at the end of its swing, so its position will vary with A. Strictly speaking, this displacement is called a *virtual* displacement: it is *as if* the gravicentre were a detached particle having the same weight as the bone and had been moved along the vertical line from where that line (drawn downwards) meets the horizontal *level* of the pendent gravicentre. This seems a very abstract way of looking at it — but all mechanical engineering depends upon it, and it works!

Geometry assures us that $h = 2r\sin^2 A/2$; and the work done against gravity is defined as wh. Hence, if E denotes this work we have:

$$(10) \quad E = 2wr \ sin^2 A/2$$

Therefore, as a bone swings (or is swung) through the range 0° to 90° to 180° so does the work done on it by the active muscles against gravity increase from 0 through wr to $2wr$.

The quantity E is the measure of the amount of energy necessary to swing the bone from the pendent position to any other position by whatever means this movement is accomplished. When the angle A is greater than that permitted by the joint at which it moves (or even when it is not greater) the swing can be supplemented by a swing of its conarticular bone at another joint. It is enough to consider the raising of a pendent bone to the antipendent position.

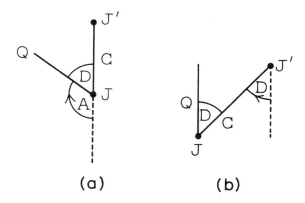

(a)   (b)

Fig. 7.6. (a) The bone Q has been swung through its maximally possible angle A from pendency (broken line) at the joint J. (b) The bone Q has been brought into antipendency by a rotation of its conarticular bone (C) through the angle D at the joint J'.

Let a bone swing through an angle A at its own joint. Then it must still be swung through an angle D in order to attain antipendency, where $D = (A-180°)$, as shown in fig. 7.6a. If its conarticular bone be then swung through this angle in the same sense as *A* (f ig. 7.6b) then the bone in question will become antipendent.

For example, if an elbow (or knee) be flexed to its maximum (143°) then a swing of the humerus (or femur) at the shoulder (or hip) will make the forearm (or leg) antipendent. The whole, fully extended, upper limb is, in fact, made antipendent by a swing of 90° of the humerus on the scapula together with swings of the scapula on the clavicle and of the clavicle on the sternum that amount to the necessary further 90°.

As the reader knows, we rarely carry out swings at single joints in our daily tasks. The work to be done, that is, the energy expended, is shared by the muscles of two or more joints in series. We know from experience how fatiguing it is to use single joints (or a series of small joints as at the fingers) repeatedly over a long time, as many specialized workers (including writers and typists!) have to do. This is why the invention of the electric typewriter, for example, has been a Godsend to one hardworking group of people: it reduces the effort that has to be made to depress the keys.

Finally, we would ask the reader to remember that it is the virtual path, not the actual path, of displacement that is the length-factor in estimating the work done and energy expended in moving a gravicentre. We shall use this principle when considering the mechanics of spin.

Spurt and Shunt Muscles

It is convenient here to define two types of muscles, the spurt and the shunt types (fig. 7.7).

i) *a spurt muscle* is one whose myonemes are all of the spurt type.

ii) *a shunt muscle* is one whose myonemes are all of the shunt type.

These names are used on the principle that a scientific term should always denote the same idea in all contexts within one and the same universe of discourse ("subject of study"). All the terms used in this book have been chosen upon this principle, whether the terms be very ancient or very modern.

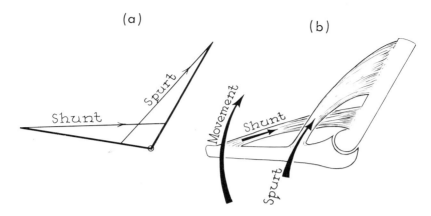

Fig. 7.7. To illustrate the concepts of spurt and shunt muscles, as described in the text. (a) a spurt fibre and a shunt fibre, (b) a spurt muscle and a shunt muscle. The arrows show the direction of pull.

The distinction between the two types will be shown later to be complete in all muscles that have a tendon at one end at least. Indeed, the only muscle that gives any rise to difficulty is the adductor magnus, whose fibres are inserted along the whole length of the shaft (*corpus*) of the femur. But even here anatomists distinguish between its upper part (*adductor quartus*) and the remainder; this upper part is the spurt portion.

The Myokinetics of Stabilization (Myostatics)

The basic myokinetics of stabilization of a bone is very easily stated. Let a bone bearing a total weight (*w*) be acted on by a total muscular force *f*, this force being that operative upon the *upper* surface of the bone. Then, if M be the moment of this force and if W be the moment of gravitational force, stabilization of the bone in one position or another of swing will occur if and only if $M = W$.

Symbols. All symbols defined already in this or the previous chapter will have the same meaning as before in all that follows.

The Radial-Ratio ρ. The ratio r/q will be very often used in both myostatics and myodynamics. It will be denoted by ρ, the Greek form of r.

It follows that for one and the same r we have $\rho'/\rho = q/q'$. This ratio ρ will be called the *radial-ratio.*

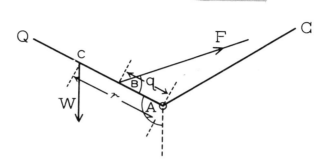

Fig. 7.8. The factors involved in the stabilization of a mobile bone (Q), articulating with a stable bone (C) in a vertical plane. W is the weight of Q acting through c, its centroid; F is the total muscular force acting upon Q at an angle B; r is the distance from c to the joint; q is the distance from the point of application of F to the joint. A is the angle between Q and a vertical line (dotted) passing towards the ground.

The Myostatic Equation: Looking at fig. 7.8 and applying equations (6, 7 and 9) we find that the mobile bone (Q in the figure) will be stabilized against gravity after a swing of $A°$ from pendency of:

(11) $M = fq \sin B = wr \sin A = 2wr \sin A/2 \cos A/2 = W$

This is the *Myostatic Equation.*

Components of Stabilizing Force. The stabilizing force (F in fig. 7.8) will have both a spurt component s and a shunt component t, the former being the stabilizing component of F.

The magnitude of s follows immediately from the equation for M:

(12) $s = f \sin B = 2w \rho \sin A/2 \cos A/2$

where ρ is the radial-ratio r/q, and q is the postaxial distance of the point of action of F. This is in fact the well-known Equation of the Lever (*levier, Hebel*), which is to often regarded as the only equation of importance in myokinetics. When $\rho > 1$, then $s > w\sin A$; when $\rho = 1$ then $s = w\sin A$; when $\rho < 1$ then $s < w\sin A$.

But the equation for t is as important as that for s on earth, moon or planet; and more important to astronauts travelling in outer space; for them, gravity cannot add its quota of safety force to that of the muscles when $A > 90°$.

Mathematics permits us to write:

$$(13) \quad t = 2wx\ \cos^2 A/2 = wx(1+\cos A)$$

In this equation x is a pure number, as yet undetermined in value; *a priori* it could be a constant or change as A changes. But even at this stage of our study we can put limits to its value. To do so we construct the equation for *total transarticular force*, denoting this by j.

$$(14) \quad j = wx(1+\cos A) - w\cos A = wx+w(x-1)\cos A$$

From this equation we see that as A changes from 0 through 90° to 180° so does j change from $w(2x-1)$ through wx to w — which is the minimal permissible value of j for an antipendent bone.

We first make $x = \frac{1}{2}$. Then for $A = 0$, $j = 0$; that is the total shunt (or safety) force is *nil*. A pendent bone would not be stable, not even metastable, but unstable; and this is biomechanically impermissible. Thus, we take $\frac{1}{2}$ as the lower limit of x.

Now make $x = 1$. In this case $j = w$ for all positions of a bone. In the case of a lower limb of a standing or sitting man w is *half* the weight of the trunk, neck, upper limbs and head. If, however, a person stands at rest on one leg (a very difficult exercise for most of us) then the load to be borne by all the joints from the hip downwards is, of course, the whole weight of the "supracoxal" part of the body together with the whole weight of the other lower limb *and also* the additional muscular components of shunt force generated by the muscles that are then active: (abductors + adductors) or (flexors + extensors). However, as these additional muscular shunt forces pull downwards, they are equivalent to an additional component of weight.

Furthermore, in standing or sitting persons the minimal total transarticular force for most bones is w, for in these people only the upper limbs are pendent; so that the scientifically modal (most common) value of j is w. We can therefore reasonably take the upper limit of x as $x = 1$.

Tentative Value of 'x.' It will be shown in myodynamics that the equation $x = 1$ is that most in accordance with the principle of muscular economy; and this value of x will be assumed to be valid in our further study of myostatics. We now proceed to draw further conclusions from equations (12) and (13).

Another Value of tanB. From the equations for s and t we find:

(15) $tanB$ = stabilization spurt-ratio = $(\rho tanA/2)/x$

(15.1) $\rho tanB = tanA/2$ if $x = 1$

Value of 'f.' From the same equations we find:

(16) $f = 2w \; cosA/2 \sqrt{\rho^2 sin^2 A/2 + x^2 cos^2 A/2}$

(16.1) $f = 2w \; cosA/2 \sqrt{\rho^2 sin^2 A/2 + cos^2 A/2}$ if $x = 1$

Hence, when $A = 180°$, $f = 0$ whatever be the value of x, for $cos\ 90° = 0$. Since all bones of a standing or sitting man are antipendent, excepting those of the upper limb, the equation satisfies the condition of minimal muscular force (except for the upper limb) even when $x = 1$; that is, it satisfies this condition for the "preferred" position of stabilization. We do not like to stand with the trunk bent forward or backward, even to a slight degree. For most bones the stabilizing force is, then, the bone's weight itself. We shall return to this matter later (see Joseph and Nightingale, 1957, for the hip).

Meanwhile, we look at the upper limb. It is shown in Chapter 8 that the weight of the whole pendent upper limb is taken by a single small muscle (supraspinatus) so disposed that it can perform this stabilizing task with a very small expenditure of energy. Again, the pendent postcubitum (forearm + hand) is close-packed with the humerus, so again we have observance of the principle of muscular economy. The hand itself has a minimum of 4 muscles to stabilize it (and any extra load) at the radio-carpal and intercarpal joints; these muscles are the carpal flexors and extensors called by that name. But a large force is necessary to stabilize either the whole limb or even the postcubitum when A lies between $0°$ and $150°$. We consider a couple of numerical examples of the postcubital stabilization, using equation (16.1).

As A passes from 0 through 90° to 180° so does f pass from 2w through $w \sqrt{2(\rho^2+1)}$ to 0. For an adult postcubitum we can take w as 2kg or 4 lb. (more or less). It is known from experiment that any one of the muscles, brachialis, biceps brachii or brachioradialis can flex the unloaded forearm acting by itself. For brachialis and biceps $\rho = 5$; and for brachioradialis $\rho = \frac{1}{2}$ (for its shorter fibres). The first two muscles are typically of the spurt kind, the third is typically a shunt muscle. For $\rho = 5f$ passes from 4kg (8 lb.) through 14 kg (28 lb.) to 0 as A changes in the way defined above. For $\rho = \frac{1}{2}f$ changes from 4kg (8 lb.) through 3.2 kg (6.4 lb.) to 0.

To judge properly the values of f given above we compare them with those f would have if it acted at right angles to the postcubitum always — the value of f assumed in the theory of levers. If this were so then f would change from 0 to 10 kg (20 lb.) again to 0 when $\rho = 5$; and from 0 to 1 kg (2 lb.) and again to 0 when $\rho = \frac{1}{2}$. We can call the values of f for $A = 90°$ the "yardstick" (comparison) values of f for that position in which gravity exerts its greatest force on a bone.

The comparison is very interesting indeed. When $\rho = 5$ the biomechanical f is 40 per cent greater than the yardstick f; but when $\rho = \frac{1}{2}$ the biomechanical value is over 300 per cent greater than the yardstick $f!$ Thus the spurt type of muscle is *relatively* more efficient as a stabilizer than a naive application of elementary lever theory would suggest. If we denote the biomechanical total force by f and the "yardstick" force by f' (= wρsinA), then we can show that

$$(17) \quad \frac{f}{f'} = \sqrt{\frac{1 + \cos^2 A/2}{\rho^2 \sin^2 A/2}} \quad (x = 1)$$

When $A = 90°$ this ratio is $(\sqrt{1+1/\rho^2})$, which is much greater when $\rho < 1$ than when $\rho > 1$; and of course, the ratio will rapidly approach 1 and as A increases from 90°. Thus for most bones in the body the actual stabilizing force is very close indeed to the engineer's ideal force. The really high values of f (in comparison with the yardstick or ideal values) are found when the whole or a part of a pendent limb is stabilized at some angle of swing between 0 and 90°; some part or all of the upper limb, or of a lower limb raised from the ground.

How often do we stand for more than a few seconds on one

leg; or with a flexed knee joint and flexed trunk, unless we are gymnasts or ballet-dancers? How often do we stand or walk with one or two upper limbs stabilized wholly or in part in some angle of flexion less than 90°? It is noteworthy that competitors in walking competitions flex their elbow joints at least to 90°, more often to more than 90°.

We have devoted much space to stabilization forces, not because we have to calculate them, but to show that the human locomotor system is much more efficient than some engineers think it is. Before proceeding to myodynamics, however, we must consider two other matters connected with stabilization. One is practical, the carriage of loads; the other is both theoretical and practical, the proof that a muscle is either a spurt or a shunt muscle according as $\rho \geqslant 1$ or $\rho < 1$, respectively.

The Carriage of External Loads. Wise men and women carry their (external) loads on their heads as much as possible, as Africans do, for example. They use that chain of antipendent bones, bifurcated below, that begins with the head, extends down the backbone and ends with the two feet. They know no kinesiology; but countless generations ago their ancestors discovered that this mode of bearing burdens was less fatiguing than carrying them by means of one or two hands; they use their arms for putting the loads on the head and for taking them off the head again. We know that this mode of bearing a burden calls for a minimal expenditure of muscular energy. But it has two other good effects also.

First, it gives a human being that upright carriage of the whole body which is a mark of human dignity. Secondly, it appears that the occurrence of ruptured intervertebral disks ("slipped disks") is much less among those who carry loads in this way than amongst those who do not.*

---

*We are grateful for this information to the orthopaedic staff of the Ghana Medical School, who have studied this matter both in their own country and in Britain, Australia, and the U.S.A.

Again, wise mothers carry their infants and young babies on the *thoracic* parts of the back, thus transferring the weight of the child directly to the chain of antipendent bones. Carrying babies on the *lumbar* part of the back is not such a good mode; it leads to a greater incidence of lumbar and lumbosacral disturbance than the thoracic mode. We are grateful to our orthopaedic colleagues in Ghana for this information also.

Finally, in this connection, it is now generally recognized that the best way to lift a load from the ground is by first bending the knees and hip joints and using the powerful muscles of the lower limbs to assist the extensor vertebral muscles to raise a slightly flexed trunk and the upper limbs. These limbs must, of course, be used to put a portable load on the head.

The Discriminant Equation. The radial-ratio ρ is more than a convenient symbol for r/q; it serves to divide muscles sharply into spurt and shunt types. To understand how it does so we consider the "effective partition-ratio" of a muscle that acts upon a bone through a tendon inserted into that bone at a postaxial distance q; this ratio (p) is that of the equivalent myoneme of all the active myonemes of the said

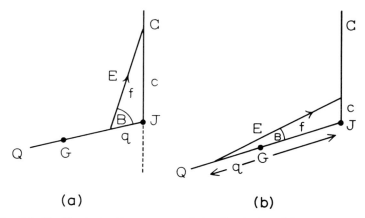

(a)   (b)

Fig. 7.9. To illustrate the concept of the Equivalent Myoneme. (a): spurt type, (b): shunt type. G is the gravicentre of the bone Q. See text.

muscle for any angle of stabilization A.

In fig. 7.9 we see two examples of such equivalent myo-nemes. In (a) $\rho > 1$ and in (b) $\rho < 1$; comparison of (a) and (b) with the spurt and shunt muscles shown in fig. 7.7 sug-gests that the first equivalent myoneme is that of a spurt muscle, the second being that of a shunt muscle. But, though diagrams may illustrate a law, they cannot prove it; proof re-quires a mathematical equation (or inequality).

For every value of A there will be a corresponding value of B, the angle of pull of the equivalent myoneme; hence a corresponding value of $tanB$. Now, we have already found two ways of expressing (or calculating) $tanB$; these are equations (4) and (15). By equating these two expressions and simplifying the resulting new equation we find:

$$(18) \quad 2cos^2A/2 = \frac{\rho(p-1)}{p(\rho-x)}$$

$$(18.1) \quad 2cos^2A/2 = \frac{\rho(p-1)}{p(\rho-1)} \text{ when } x = 1$$

These are the general and the special forms of *The Discrim-inant Equation.*

Take the special form first. It shows that if $\rho \geqslant 1$ then $p \geqslant 1$; if $\rho < 1$ then $p < 1$. This is because $cos^2A/2$ is never negative, so that $(\rho-1)$ and $(p-1)$ must each be either negative or posi-tive (or both zero). Thus *all spurt myonemes must be inserted nearer to the swing-axis of a joint than the gravicentre of an externally unloaded bone; and all shunt myonemes must be inserted further from the said gravicentre than this latter's distance from the said axis.* This is why the equation (18.1) is called "discriminant."

In equation (18) x could be of any value between ½ and 1, as we saw when considering equation (14). This merely al-ters the value of the "discriminator" (x). As already stated we shall take $x = 1$ for the time being.

The discriminating equation is valid if and only if both B and p change with A. Thus we cannot use it:

i) If the muscle has also a tendon (or a very small area) of origin; for then p is constant.

ii) If B changes very little with A (as in the deltoid).

The equation applies in fact to those muscles, such as the triangular kind, in which successive bundles of myonemes can be brought into action as A changes. Thus it applies to the brachialis and brachioradialis but not to either head of the biceps brachii; and it applies to the short head but not to the long head of the biceps femoris.

Nevertheless, the rule that $p \geqslant 1$ and $p < 1$ according as $\rho \geqslant 1$ and $\rho < 1$, respectively, does apply to all muscles with one exception. The exception is the middle part of the deltoid, which never acts by itself (in normal folk) but always as a powerful assistant prime mover in conjunction with the supraspinatus. This part of deltoid is of the shunt type anatomically; functionally it is an extension of the upper part of the trapezius that acts with it in abduction of the whole upper limb beyond 90°.

Summary of Myostatic Results

Before we proceed to myodynamics it is advisable to summarize the chief results of our study of myostatics. They are as follows:

1) As a bone of weight w passes from pendency to antipendency so does the force needed to stabilize it securely against gravity changes from a maximum of $2w$ to 0. This is the total muscular force, not merely its spurt component.

2) There is a one-to-one correspondence between this total force and the angle through which the bone is swung before being stabilized.

3) There is a one-to-one correspondence between the angle (A) at which stabilization is effected and the angle at which the total muscular force acts on the bone. This latter angle (B) never exceeds 90°.

4) The division of muscles into a spurt type and a shunt type is supported by the theory of stabilization.

5) If a certain factor x has the value 1 then the total trans-articular force along the bone is equal to the weight of the bone for all values of A (3, above); this force being generated by the combined actions of gravity and of the total muscular force.

Antigravitational Myodynamics of Swing

When a bone swings through an angle A from some position of stabilization, denoted by an angle A', it does so at a rate a (radians or degrees per second). As it swings the angle of application of the force required (B) will also change, because of the one-to-one correspondence between B and A. The change in B is the cause of the change in A; denoting the rate of change in B (in radians or degrees per second) by b; we say, therefore, that b is the cause of a. The relation between the two is a/b.

Clearly, the chief problem in myodynamics is to find the relation between a/b and the force f which is the cause of b. This force is the *myodynamic force*.

It has long been known experimentally that muscular action is continuous during a swing (or spin). Muscles have to act continuously against gravity because the momentum of a bone caused by an initial force applied to it is never enough to make it move "on its own" like a projectile fired from a gun — the so-called "ballistic" hypothesis. Thus, f will have some definite value at each instant of swing, this instant being defined by the angle A at that moment.

We begin by considering motion against gravity. After that we consider the relation between b and activity of the motor neurones of the nervous system. This is a necessary preliminary to understanding the synergic part played by muscles when a motion is downward, gravity being then the prime mover.

The Relation of 'a' to 'b'. The ratio of a/b to the instantaneous value of A will be stated without proof, for it requires the differential calculus to determine it. The factor x in the equation now to be given is that which was left undetermined in our myostatic studies. From the equation given in the foot-note* we find:

$$(19) \quad \frac{a}{b} = \frac{2x \cos^2 A/2}{\rho \cos^2 B}$$

The equation for a/b will now be explained (fig. 7.10). The upward swing of a bone is due to the fact that at any instant the moment M of the total force is greater than M', the moment needed for stability, so that $(M-W)>0$, where W is the gravitational moment. Now, both a and b are independent of whether the bone starts from stability or is moving; we

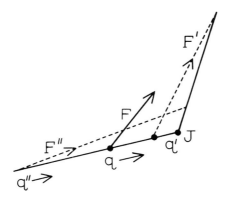

Fig. 7.10. A spurt force F' and a shunt force F" are equivalent conjointly to a single force F that acts on a bone further from J than F' acts.

---

*Denoting time by t (for this equation only), we have $a = dA/dt$ and $b = dB/dt$. The differential equation is:

$$\frac{dA}{dt} = \frac{dA}{d(A/2)} \cdot \frac{d(A/2)}{d\tan A/2} \cdot \frac{d\tan A/2}{d\tan B} \cdot \frac{d\tan B}{dB} \cdot \frac{dB}{dt}$$

The solution given in the text follows from the fact that $\tan B = (\rho \tan A/2)/x$ as was shown in myostatics. The factor x is assumed to be constant.

can, therefore, assume it to be stable to begin with. The equivalent myoneme (F in the figure) then exercises a moment M' and a corresponding stabilizing force f'. Since M is fixed all that is necessary for F to do is to increase f' by an amount $(f-f')$ to the myodynamic force f.

If the *principle of muscular economy* is to be observed then only the *spurt* component of f' needs to be increased, for this is both necessary and sufficient to increase M' to M. We can therefore write for any value of A:

$$(20) \quad f\cos B = f'\cos B = 2wx\cos^2 A/2$$

From equations (19) and (20) we can now determine four things:

    i) The "acceptable" value of x.

    ii) The minimal value of f.

    iii) The variation of a/b with ρ.

The value of x and 'f'. By multiplying the right-hand side of equation (19) by $(f/f)^2$ $(=1)$, remembering the value of $f\cos B$ given in equation (20) and reducing the resulting equation to its simplest terms we find:

$$(21) \quad a = \frac{2\,b\,f^2}{\rho x\,(2w\,\cos A/2)^2}$$

It follows that a will be minimal for a given (b, f, ρ, w and A) if x be maximal. But what would this mean physically?

Action. In the mechanical order of things f produces b and b produces a. At any moment, then, the bone will possess a certain kinetic energy (k), whose amount is $w\ r^2a^2/2g$, as is shown in physics; here g is the local constant of gravitational acceleration.

In the earlier part of this century it was found necessary to introduce a new quantity into basic physics. This quantity is called *Action* and is defined as the product of energy by time (energy × time). If a bone swings for t seconds and has a kinetic energy k then it does so because its Action is of an amount kt. This is a definition of *osteokinetic action.*

Muscular Power. The term *power* has a precise meaning in physics: it means the rate at which some mechanism carries out a particular piece (or quantity) of work, as this term has been defined earlier (p. 148). Thus if the acting musculature causes a swing of $A°$ (from pendency) over a time t, then its power is E/t, where E is the work done on the gravicentre of the bone swung by the musculature.

We shall now see how the concept of the power of an acting muscle mass leads to the concept of Action.

Work-Action Ratio. Let a bone be swung from pendency through an angle A over a time t at an average rate of swing a. Then we have at once:

$$(22.1) \quad \frac{\text{Muscular Power}}{\text{Kinetic Energy}} = \frac{E/t}{k} = \frac{E}{kt} = \frac{\text{Work done on bone}}{\text{Action involved}}$$

Since $E = 2\ wr\ sin^2A/2$ and $k = w\ r^2a^2/2g$, we have:

$$(22.2) \quad E/kt = (4g\ sin^2A/2)/rt\ a^2 = \text{work-action ratio}$$

Now the work is done by the musculature; and it follows that this work accomplished by muscular effort is maximal relative to the Action imparted to the bone by the musculature if a is minimal; that is, if x is maximal.

We have seen that it is both necessary and sufficient if $x = 1$ when $A = 180°$; and that this value of x is sufficient if the bones are to be kept in contact during stabilization. Hence we take 1 as the "acceptable" maximal value of x; for this leads to a minimal quantity of Action per unit of work done against gravity. We therefore write:

$$(23) \quad f = 2\ w\ cos\ A/2\ \sqrt{\frac{pa}{2b}}$$

It will now be shown that f is the minimal force required for motion against gravity.

The Variation of (a/b) with ρ. The ratio of angular speed is closely related to both the radial-ratio ρ of the total muscular force, and also to the instantaneous angle of position (A) of the moving bone.

From equation (19), taking $x = 1$ as we now must do, we find:

$$a/b = \frac{2cos^2A/2}{\rho\ cos^2B}$$

Now, $1/(cos^2B) = 1+tan^2B = \rho^2tan^2A/2+1$ (since $x = 1$) Hence:

(24) $a/b = \dfrac{2}{\rho}(cos^2A/2 + \rho^2sin^2A/2) = (2^2cos^2A/2)/\rho 2\rho\ sin^2A/2$

Both expressions for a/b have their special uses. From either of them we see that as A changes from 0 through 90° to 180° so does a change from $2b/\rho$ through $b/(1/\rho + \rho)$ to $2\rho\ b$.

It follows that for any *constant* value of b —

i) A *spurt* muscle (or set of muscles) will produce a rate of swing that will be slow to begin with and then become more and more rapid.

ii) A *shunt* muscle will produce a rate of swing that will be rapid to begin with and then become increasingly slow.

iii) The rate of swing will be constant if $\rho = 1$.

iv) If ρ is not 1 then the rate of swing will be constant if b changes as A changes; though in a mathematically complex way. How this happens in fact will be studied in the next section of this chapter.

Let us take three numerical examples. In all of these $b = 10°$ per second.

i) If $\rho = 1$, then $a = 20°$ per sec., a slow rate.

ii) If $\rho = 5$ (spurt type) then a will change from 4° through 52° to 100° per second.

iii) If $\rho = ½$ (shunt type) then a will change from 40° through 25° to 10° per second.

These examples illustrate the fact that spurt muscles are very suitable for slow motions — and, in the limbs, for stabilization — when A lies in the range 0° to 90°.

The magnitude of the myodynamic force. Before finding the magnitude of the myodynamic swing-force f we recall a fact that may seem at first to be too obvious to merit being mentioned: *Motion of a bone is produced by continued contraction of its musculature; and stabilization occurs when contraction is replaced by simple hardening of the operative myonemes.*

We now find the value of f by taking equation (23) and substituting for a/b in this equation the first of the expressions for a/b in equation (24). The result is:

$$(25) \quad f = 2wcos A/2\sqrt{\rho^2sin^2A/2 + cos^2A/2}$$

But, you may say, that is the equation for the stabilizing force for any given w, ρ and A. Precisely; it is! The equation is the mathematical equivalent of the statement that was emphasized in the preceding paragraph. Because of the one-to-one relationship between the stabilizing force on the one hand, and the "triple set" of factors (w, ρ and A) on the other hand it is both necessary and sufficient for the swing-force to be equal to the stabilizing force; that is, if the principle of muscular economy is to operate. Let us examine this statement —

i) The myodynamic force required for a swing against gravity cannot be less than the stabilizing force; for if it were less then the swing would be downwards, not upwards.

ii) For the same reason the *minimal* swing force cannot be greater than the stabilizing force; for if it were it would be greater than is both necessary and sufficient, and so not minimal.

All that is necessary to produce a swing is, then, a continuing change in the angle (B) between the bone and the total force vector acting on it. Before inquiring into how this change is caused we must look at a third component of the transarticular force that is present in a moving bone.

The Newtonian Transarticular Force

Some 300 years ago Isaac Newton made certain assumptions (postulates) about the forces acting upon moving bodies and he explained the curvilinear motions of moons and planets upon the basis of a centripetal force acting continuously upon the moving body and directed towards that centre of the "fixed" body. His arithmetic had to be modified by Einstein at the beginning of our century, but it was nevertheless very successful in helping to build up the science of astronomy.

Today we know that this centripetal force is always present when a body moves in a curved path. But it can be *an effect* not the cause of that motion; furthermore it can (and does) exist as a supplement to any centripetal force that is present when the body is at rest. This is true of our bones. When they are at rest there is a *static centripetal force* acting along them towards their joints; but when they are moving this is increased by a Newtonian (*dynamic*) centripetal force, which varies as the square of the rate of swing (in the present context), that is, as a^2. This force we shall denote by n for an obvious reason.

The curvilinear path of the bones is not the result of n; it is due to the fact that the moving articular surface of a bone is pressed towards its conarticular joint surface by the co-existing static centripetal force generated by gravity and/or the active myonemes. In other words, n is the result of the curved motion of the bone, not the cause of it; and *no additional muscular force is needed to produce it.* This is proved in Appendix C.*

But although n is not produced by an additional musculo-gravitational shunt force, yet it has a relation to the spurt force whose continued action produces the motion. This is the reason why we have to consider it.

First we write the equation for n. It has been known since Newton's time that:

$$(25) \quad n = wra^2/g$$

Here g is the local acceleration (increase of speed per second)

---

*The proof, though very simple, requires the use of vector algebra. It is an improved form of that first used by MacConaill (1957).

of any corporeal body falling freely towards the centre of our Earth, our moon or a planet; this is 32 ft. per second per second (or 981 cm per sec per sec) for mid-Northern or mid-Southern latitudes of our Earth.

The Newtonian component of transarticular force is, then, dependent upon w, r and a^2. For any particular values of these quantities it has a specific value at any instant during motion. It is therefore a useful "yardstick" (comparison) force by which to measure s, the spurt component of the total muscular force at that instant. Since s is the spurt component of the stabilizing force at that instant, then, taking n as the unit for measuring s, we have:

$$(26) \quad \frac{s}{n} = \frac{w\rho \sin A}{wra^2/g} = \frac{g \sin A}{qa^2}$$

The only "choice" (for a given n) is q; where q is the postaxial distance of the point at which s acts. As q increases, so does s decrease and f decrease (because $f\cos B$ is fixed for a given A). Since we can write s as $(ng\sin A)/qa^2$, we can call equation (26) the *Law of the Living Lever*. It agrees with the law of the "dead lever" in that s varies inversely as q, other things being equal (*caeteris paribus*). Let us look at a couple of numerical examples.

Suppose that $a = 1$ radian ($57°$) per second and $A = 90°$. Then f/n is g/q. The factors q and g must each be stated in feet or centimetres; but the retio g/q is the same in each case. If $q = \frac{1}{2}$inch ($=1/24$ feet $= 1.27$ cm) then $s = 768n$. If $q = 12$ inches then $s = 32n$. Hence as q passes from 0.5 inches (1.27 cm) to 12 inches (nearly 30.7 cm) so does s decrease in value to 1/64 of its initial value. If the bone be the postcubitum then the first q is that appropriate to the brachialis and biceps brachii, the second q is that appropriate to the brachioradialis; the three being potentially flexors of the forearm.

The motor spurt force is, then, proportional to a^2 and therefore to n. If a is large then it is reasonable to expect that shunt musculature will be called in to assist any spurt musculature being used, for the purpose of economy of muscular effort; because this will lengthen the virtual (or effective) length of q.

This is illustrated in fig. 7.10 which shows (though not to scale) how a spurt force F′ and a shunt force F″ are together equivalent to a force F that acts at a postaxial distance q greater than that (q') at which the spurt force acts.

This reinforcement of a spurt musculature by a shunt musculature is invariable at the shoulder during pure abduction or during swings involving some abduction. At rest the whole upper limb is stabilized by the spurt-type supraspinatus (see Chapter 8); but during motion the shunt-type deltoid is always called into action to assist the supraspinatus; for f is always large in a moving whole upper limb, that is, in terms of n.

Again, the q of a multiarticular muscle is always longer (with respect to the joint nearest to the point from which it pulls) than if it were a uniarticular muscle. In this fact may lie the explanation of the occurrence of the multiarticular type in cases where a uniarticular type would seem sufficient. In this connection one may mention the two parts of the triceps surae, the muscular mass that pulls the heelbone (calcaneus) upwards. Its gastrocnemial part has a much longer q than its soleal part, and it is always used in running and jumping.

Finally, and not least important, is the fact that for a given bone moving at some particular speed, n is the same whether the swing be in a clockwise or an anticlockwise sense. Hence the bringing into action of *one and the same shunt muscle* during rapid motion in both, say, flexion and extension, is to be expected — provided that this does not involve the use of otherwise unnecessary synergic muscles. The brachioradialis is one of the muscles that can be used in this way. It is used in flexion of the elbow and in stabilization when the load to be moved or stabilized is large. But it is active in both flexion and extension when these are rapid (Basmajian, 1959), because n increases as the square of the speed; and as the rate of swing of the elbow joint increases from 57° per sec to 114° per sec and more, so does n increase to 4 times its value (not twice), and from a certain value through 4 times that value and then 16 times that value as a

increases from 28°, through 57° to 114° per sec.

Why a flexor muscle should be used in extension at all will be shown in the section following the next one. But it is certainly economical to do so!

A Basic Neurokinesiology

First, it should be noted that the word "neurone" will denote a motor neurone in all that follows. Every myone is the slave of its neurone; and every myoneme is therefore the slave of the set of neurones that acts upon its myones. Look at fig. 7.11. It shows a linear series of three myones, M, M' and M''; each myone having its private neurone N, N' and N'', respectively. Accoring to whether we have N or (N + N') or (N + N' + N'') in action so *must* M or (M + M') or (M + M' + M'') come into action also.

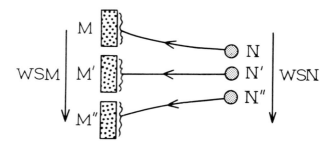

Fig. 7.11. A sequence of neurones (or sets of neurones) N, N', N'', acts on a sequence of myones (or sets of myones) M, M', M''. WSN, wave of stimulation of neurones. WSM, wave of stimulation of myones. See text.

Look at the figure again. This time M, M' and M'' each represent a linear *set* of myones, part of a myoneme in fact; and N, N' and N'' each represents a linear set of neurones, part of a motor "cell-column" within the nervous system, in fact. For

brevity we shall speak of the "M-series" and the "N-series."
There are two ways in which the M-series can be made to
act —

i) *Statically:* in this form of action the N-series sends impulses *simultaneously* so rapidly to the whole M-series that
   the myones cannot relax and so remain hardened. This is
   obviously the neural basis of myostatics.

ii) *Kinematically:* in this form of action the neurones of the
    N-series čome into action one after another and so the
    members of the M-series come into action successively,
    thus causing contraction (shortening) of the myoneme.
    This is obviously the neural basis of myokinematics.

The Rate of Muscular Contraction. When neurones act kinematically they do so because they are brought into action
by a *wave of stimulation;* this wave may start at one or other
end of an N-series, or spread in both directions through it.
The important thing is that it will have a certain speed of
travel.

Reference to fig. 7.11 will show that the speed of travel of
the "neuronic" wave must also be that of the "myonic"
wave, after a certain delay depending on the length of the
motor nerves that transmit the neuronic wave. Hence in muscles unaffected by disease or drugs *the speed of contraction
of muscles will be the speed of the neuronic wave that produces the contraction.*

It is for this reason that it is sufficient for the total spurt
force of acting musculature to be that of the stabilizing force
at any instant for motion to take place as the result of modi-
fication of the state of activity within the central nervous system. Because of the one-to-one relation of the total muscle
force to the total angle of swing, all that is required to swing
a bone from one position to another is to change this force to
one appropriate to the intended new position. Kinetically
the thing is very simple indeed.

The complexity lies within that extraordinarily complicated
computer that rules our muscles from within the skull and the
backbone. To make its actions understandable is the task of
the neurophysiologists, a most industrious nation. But not

even the most distinguished of them has any knowledge of the exact way in which his (or her) own computer is "programmed" to perform even the simplest action. It is true that some people can be trained to bring into action one and only one of the neurones of some identifiable group. But they cannot choose which particular neurone of that group is to be the servant of their will.

The Skilled and the Clumsy. The fact is that we learn how to control the action of our musculature (*not* of our individual muscles) from infancy onwards by a process of trial and error; correcting the errors by further experiments until what we do arouses in us the desired feelings (*sensibilité, Empfehlung*). These feelings are caused by a multitude of sensory impulses coming from the muscles themselves, from the joints, from our eyes and other appropriate sensory organs. Those who achieve a good control of their muscles we call "skilled," the others we call "clumsy."

But in reality it is the motor neuronic system that we learn to control. All human kinesiology depends on the last analysis upon events in the nervous system — *nervi domini musculi servi* — the nerves are the masters, the muscles are their slaves.

Gravitational Swing

We already know the weight of a bone is a force constant in direction — which is why work done against it is measured with respect to a vertical line. This force is that normally used by us for extending and/or adducting bones; it is the only inexhaustible source of energy there is. But it is always modified in strength, never allowed to act alone; for if it did the bone would move faster and faster and the joint would be in danger of a violent dislocation, as we know, not only by the gravitational shunt component but also by its spurt component.

It is now well established experimentally that when gravity

is the prime mover in a swing then some part of the antigravitational swing musculature is operative to determine the actual rate of swing, for example, to make it slow or fast at a
constant rate. This active musculature is a *synergist* to gravity, not an antagonist. This is a matter of the degree of force
exercised by it; if the degree were great enough, then the
said musculature would be fully antagonist in its action and
stabilize the bone. Sometimes, indeed, down-pulling muscles are used to *augment* the force of gravity; as in stamping
a foot violently on the ground, or in pressing part of the upper
limb downwards against some external resistance. But even
in these cases synergic antigravitational musculature is also
operative.

Apart from the need to prevent the joint from being dislocated, the use of the synergic (or even augmentatory) musculature fulfils another biological purpose: *it brings the motor
action of gravity under the control of the nervous system.* It
is b, in this case the speed of lessening of the angle (B) made
by the synergic muscle and the bone, that again determines
the magnitude of a, now the downward rate of swing; and, as
we have seen, b is determined by the motor neurones, though
in a complex way.

We can now see why a flexor muscle like the brachioradialis should be active during rapid extension of the elbow. It
helps to proportion the force of the synergic flexor musculature to the Newtonian centripetal force associated with a
high rate of swing upwards or downwards; and to do this in
accordance with the principle of muscular economy.

The Myokinetics of Spin

Excepting one case to be discussed later, gravity plays no
part in spin movement. Nevertheless, the weight of a bone,
here taken as a measure of its mass, is of primary importance.
This weight involves the amount of work done by the musculature in producing a given angle of spin, whether or not the
spin can be produced independently of a swing (as at the

shoulder and hip joints) or is dependent upon the amount of swing (as at all other joints).

In this connection it must be mentioned that the work done in producing a given amount of swing is the same whether the spin be produced by an arcuate motion or by a diadochal motion. This follows from the principle of "the separability of variables" without which physics would be impossible.

When studying the myokinetics of spin we use not only the concept of the equivalent myoneme but also that of an *equivalent disk*. This latter concept plays the same part in the kinetics of spin as does the gravicentre in the kinetics of swing.

In physics it is shown that, when we consider the kinetics of a rod that is rotated (spun) around its long axis then the rod can be replaced by a disk that fulfils two conditions:

i) The disk has the weight of the rod and any load that rotates as the rod itself rotates:

ii) The disk is perpendicular (normal) to the rod's long axis, and is placed transversely to the rod at the level of operation of the force-vector of spin; this vector is a tangent to the rim (boundary) of the disk.

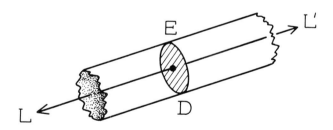

Fig. 7.12. The Equivalent Disk (ED) of a bone. Only part of the bone is shown. LL', longitudinal axis of the bone in the region of the disk. See text.

A disk fulfilling these conditions in the case of a bone is an *equivalent disk* of that bone. The reader is referred to fig. 7.12, in which such a disk is shown; but only a part of the bone is shown in the figure.*

The mechanics of spin is very simple (fig. 7.13). We take an equivalent myoneme E which passes transversely around a bone (therefore transversely around the equivalent disk) to be attached to some appropriate point on the rim of the

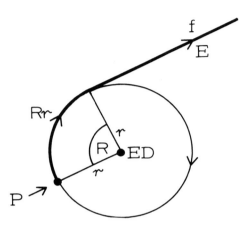

Fig. 7.13. The gyrovial equivalent myoneme (E) is attached at the point P to the periphery of an equivalent disk ED. By contracting through a distance Rr, E spins the disk (and the bone) through an angle R. The myoneme exercises an average force f over the distance Rr.

disk. Let the radius of the disk be r and its weight (that of the whole bone) be w. As E contracts through a distance Rr, so will the disk rotate through an angle R around the bone's long axis.

─────────

*Physicists and engineers refer to spin as "torsion," and to a spin-force as a "torsional force." In biomechanics, certainly in biomedical mechanics, to use the word *torsion* would be confusing. The word itself means "twisting" and medical people quite correctly say that bones can be fractured by torsion — a very common accident when a bone is brought suddenly and violently into close-pack with another. But no bone is ever broken by spin *per se:* to cause fracture one end of the bone must be held rigidly, so that this end does not spin. We have chosen all our kinematic and kinetic terms very carefully, both here and in our earlier scientific papers, in such a way as to lessen the possibility of confusion by an ambiguous use of physical terms.

During its contraction the myoneme will use a total amount of energy fRr, where f is the *average* force per angle of spin. This energy is equal to the amount of work done by the myoneme in causing the disk to spin through the angle R. It appears from physics that the amount of this work is $(8wr\ sin^2R/2)/3\pi^2$. It follows that:

$$(27)\quad f = \frac{8w\ sin^2R/2}{3\pi^2R}\quad (3\pi^2 = 30\text{ very nearly})$$

This is the *force-equation* of spin.

It is to be noted that the spin-force is independent of the radius, unlike a swing-force. It is also to be noted that the weight w is that of the whole part of the body that is rotated by a spin. Thus it is the weight of the whole upper or lower limb in rotation of a humerus or femur, as the case may be. In the case of pronation or supination it is the weight of the postcubitum, and of any load carried by the hand and/or of any external resistance to the movement — for a resistance is equivalent to a weight.

The equation (27) gives the *minimal* average force of the gyrovial element of a motion. This force will be that exerted by the radio-ulnar part of the supinator in supination by that muscle alone. But the force to be exerted will increase with the degree of obliquity of an arcuival muscle. The more transverse muscles passing to the humerus (e.g., subscapularis) and to the femur (e.g. internal obturator) are largely gyrovial in their action in contrast to the more chordovial deltoid and psoas muscles, respectively.

Swing versus Spin. The best comparison of the kinetics of swing and of spin for any one bone is that between the amount of work done by the musculature in causing either a swing or a spin through one and the same angle. Denote this angle by A in each case; and let r' be the radius of the part of the bone to which the total spin force is applied, r being the distance from the axis of swing to the bone's gravicentre. Then, from the data respecting work done by spin forces given in this section and equation (10), we find:

$$(28) \quad \frac{e}{E} = \frac{4r'}{3\pi r}$$

Here e is the work done by the spin force and E is that done by the swing force. The equation makes it clear that both the weight of the bone and the angle of spin or swing are irrelevant to the ratio of the work done.

Take a postcubitum as an example. If no weight be carried in the hand, then 15 cm is a typical adult value of r and 1 cm is the corresponding average value of r' taken along the part of the radius that receives the muscles of pro-supination. The ratio e/E is therefore $4/45\pi$, that is, $1/35$; in words, 35 times as much work must be done by the antibrachial swing muscles (in swinging a postcubitum through any angle) as is done by the pronator or supinator muscles in turning the hand through the same angle.

We can go further and say: *For one and the same angle of motion the work to produce a spin of that angle is always less than the work done to produce a swing of the same amount.* For if the work done in each case were the same then we should have $r' = 3\pi r/4 = 2.35r$. This is true for no bone in the body, r being usually much greater than r'.

Gravity as a Spin Force. There is an important exception to the rule that gravity usually does not generate a spin. It is found in the upper limb.

Abduct (or flex) an upper limb through 90° and then flex its forearm through an angle E (fig. 7.14). As the figure shows, the weight of the forearm (w) acting downwards through the antebrachial gravicentre (at a distance r from the flexion-axis) will exert a spin-moment $wr \sin E$ upon the humerus. When E = 90° then this moment is maximal, being then wr. If the angle of flexion and/or abduction of the humerus be B, then the spin-moment will be $wr \sin E \sin B$; maximal when $B = E = 90°$.

Thus to maintain a given level of elevation of a flexed forearm some part of the *lateral rotator* musculature of the shoulder joint must come into action as an anti-spin stabilizer. The posterior part of the deltoid muscle will often be

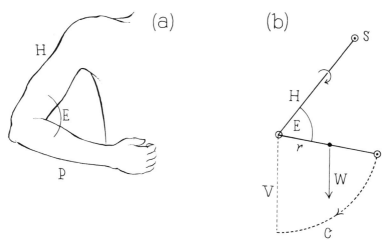

Fig. 7.14. To illustrate rotational effect of a postcubitum (P) upon a humerus (H) that has been abducted through a right angle. The Elbow has been flexed through an angle E. (a) shows position of humerus and postcubitum; (b) shows the mechanical scheme: *r*, distance from centre of elbow joint to centroid of postcubitum through which the postcubital weight (W) acts, generating a rotational force acting on the humerus at the centre of the shoulder joint (S); the direction of the rotation is shown by the small curved arrow. The dotted line (V) is vertical. C (curved dotted line) shows the direction in which the postcubitum would move if suitable musculature at the shoulder were not operative.

enough for this purpose; for the medial spin to be prevented would stretch this part of the muscle. If, however, the angle E and/or B were less than 45°, then the teres minor could well be sufficient, unless the hand were carrying a load of, say 2 lbs. (or 1 kg).

Palmar flexion or dorsiflexion of the hand in an otherwise extended and abducted upper limb would have a similar effect but to a much less degree.

The Speed of Spins. Let a be the rate per second of change of R, that is, of the speed of a spin. Then reference to fig. 7.14 will show that a is precisely the rate of change (shortening) of the length Rr. This, in turn, is precisely the rate of the neuronic wave of stimulation of the neurones that supply the linear sets of myones involved. Here again, then, but more

directly, we see that the speed of a movement is wholly dependent upon the central nervous system.

But, since rapid speed of spin demands the expenditure of
more energy per second than does a slow speed, we should
expect that additional spin musculature would be brought
into use in rapid spins — if available. This has been verified
for pronation and supination (see Chapter 8).

Weight-Bearing and Joints

In times past, even sometimes today, certain quite good
anatomists have talked about "the weight-bearing position"
of a joint. They have even tried to define it for different
joints! In plain scientific language, the term is pure nonsense.

The common experience, that is, the commonsense of man-
kind over some 200,000 years has shown that a joint can
bear weight in *any* of its possible positions. Some positions
are more comfortable than others; some are more uncom-
fortable, even painful: but that does not affect the issue. For
so long as a weight does not dislocate a joint then the joint
bears the weight. *There is no unique weight-bearing position
of a joint.*

There are, however, weight-bearing positions of parts of
the body that are maximally economical of muscular energy.
For the upper limbs *as a whole* the position is that of pendency; for all other parts it is the position of antipendency.
We have looked at these positions in detail above. Again excepting the upper limb, all antipendent joints are near, but
not exactly in, the position of maximal congruency — of close-
pack. In the nearly-congruent position, the deformability of
articular cartilage has the effect of reducing the pressure
caused by weight (and other forces) across a joint to the low
level associated with full congruency — but without the danger associated with close-pack, which is a statistically exceptional position.

With respect to the elbow we would emphasize that in man
(but not in all animals) there are *two* joints (articular units)

in which the humerus and ulna take part. One is the *olecrano-humeral*, whose position of close-pack is that of full extension. The other is the *coronoido-humeral*, whose close-packed position is at or near 90° of flexion. If the radius then be semi-pronated it also is maximally congruent with the capitular surface of the humerus; so that then we have *full antebrachial congruence with the humerus.* The two parts of the humeral surface of the ulna are usually separated by a narrow, transverse, *non-articular* region covered by synovial membrane — which *never* bears weight. The position of full antebrachial congruence is for hitting something — or somebody; the position of olecrano-humeral close-pack is excellent for beginning a pull on something — or somebody.

The myth of "the weight-bearing position of a joint" comes down to us from the scientists of the Atlantic mid-Victorian culture. They carried no burden on their heads except their top-hats; and thought themselves superior to those who carried other burdens on their heads, particularly as these latter folk had not retained the lack of pigmentation (of skin, hair and eyes) of the embryo. They had a strange notion that human upper limbs were for holding things instead of for moving things from one place to another — from platters to mouths or from the ground to the tops of heads. And, although evolution was their God and Darwin was his Prophet, they had a marked disposition to point out what imperfect and dangerous things were the upright backbone and the bipedal position. We still have some of that tribe with us today. They are less vocal.

One of the many myths of the 19th century was transmitted to it by Newton, who was compelled to invent it. It is that of "action at a distance." We know better now; even gravitation has a wave-length! For this reason we were interested to find that the principle of muscular economy in the myokinetics of swing led to the consequence that the total transarticular force was equal to that of the total load of and upon a bone stabilized at its joint; plus the non-Newtonian (or strictly, generalized Newtonian) force transmitted to the joint during motion of the swing type. In other words, every position of a joint is one of full weight-bearing. Of course, when a person stands with both feet on the ground, then the "weight" borne by each lower limb, from the hip joint downwards, is half of the total weight of the head, trunk and upper limbs.

That the total weight borne by successively lower parts of an erect man is transferred through joint after joint to the ground (where the feet make contact with it) is obvious; except in the case of the two upper limbs and that of a lower limb raised from the ground. The physical problem posed by the exceptions (and by a trunk bent forwards or backwards in a standing or sitting man) can be put in the form of a question: *How can the vertical force we call the weight of a part of the body, and acting through the gravicentre of that part, be transferred to one or both lower limbs and so to the ground without the involvement of action at a distance?*

The answer to the question is provided by a fundamental physical principle, namely, that of Virtual Rotation of Vectors.

The Principle of Virtual Rotation. If a vector acting in some initial direction be first rotated through an angle A and be then rotated through an equal and opposite angle $(-A)$ it then will *either* act in its original direction and through the same point; *or* it will act through some other point in a direction *parallel to* its initial direction. Since vectors are not material objects any of the rotations described above must be a *virtual rotation.*

Application of the Principle. Let the reader refer to fig. 7.15. In (a) is shown the weight (W) of a limb acting through the limb's gravicentre G. The limb makes contact with the trunk at the joint J; the trunk is represented for simplicity by the vertical line labelled T in (b) of the figure; T makes contact with the ground (HH′) through one or both lower limbs. The problem is, then: how can the weight-vector W be "transferred" to T, so that it acts vertically downwards through T and so reaches the ground where it can affect, say, a weighing-machine? In (a) the "transferred W" is represented by W″.

The first stage of the solution of the problem is shown in (b) of the figure. The spurt-effect of W is nullified by suitable muscular spurt forces applied to the limb. At the same instant suitable muscular shunt forces supplement the shunt-

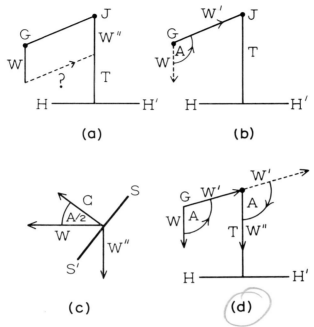

Fig. 7.15. To illustrate the "transference" of the weight (W) of a bone from the gravicentre G to the trunk T at the joint J. Full details in text.

(a) The problem. (b) The first virtual rotation of W. (c) The components of the reactive force (-W′) at the joint surface. (d) The second virtual rotation of W. SS′: part of the surface of the scapula; G is the gravicentre of the humerus in this case.

effect of W in such a way that the total shunt force acting along the limb towards J is equal in magnitude to W. Thus *in effect* W has been virtually rotated into the limb through the angle *A*; if the rotated W be denoted by W′, as in the figure, *A* is the angle between W and W′.

The second stage, that of the equal and opposite virtual rotation of W, takes place at the conarticular surface of the bone into which W has been "rotated." When the force W′ acts on this surface, as shown in (c) of fig. 7.15, an equal and opposite *reactive force* (-W′) is generated; this is one of the basic postulates of mechanics, first stated by Newton and so far not disproved by experiment. Newton went no further, being interested mainly in celestial mechanics. We must go further, for we are interested in biomechanics.

As is shown in (c) of the figure, the reactive force (-W′) can be, and is, resolved into two components. One is a *vertical* component W″ equal in magnitude to W and parallel with it. The other component (C) makes an angle $A/2$ with the reactive force itself and has a magnitude $2w \cos^2 A/2$. We are not concerned with C for it has itself a multitude of small components which are nullified by the counter-stresses set up within the articular cartilage, particularly its non-fibrous parts.

Of the existence of the vertical, downward-acting component W″ there is no doubt whatever. Its existence is verified every time a person has his or her weight recorded by a weighing-machine. In particular, if a previously weighted object be taken into that person's hand, its weight will be added to that recorded by the weighing machine.

The generation of W″ and the intra-cartilaginous (or possibly intra-osseal) nullification of C are together equivalent to a virtual rotation of W′ through an angle -A within the bone that receives the total transarticular force, as shown in (d) of the figure. But this, in turn, is equivalent to a virtual rotation of W through an angle A, followed by its transference to another bone, followed by its virtual counter-rotation into a line parallel with its initial line of action. This proves the theorem.

Generalization of the Application. It is clear that what has just been proved for the upper limb (humerus) in relation to the trunk (scapula) is applicable to all joints within a limb or other part of the body. For example, the weight of a loaded or unloaded hand is transferred along its bones to the wrist-joint, where it becomes part of the weight of the forearm; the other part being the weight of the forearm itself. At the elbow joint the weight of the whole postcubitum becomes part of the weight of the arm; and so on. Similarly the several weights of the parts of a lower limb raised off the ground, beginning with the weight of the foot, are successively transferred *in toto* to the pelvis of that side to the trunk; and are transferred to the ground *via* the other lower limb.

What we have now done is to abolish any distinction between the joints of antipendent bones and those of non-anti-
pendent bones as bearers of the total weight of the parts of
the body which, directly or indirectly, move or are stabilized
at them. All our weight is generated by the centripetal pull
of the earth, moon or planet on which we are. It returned to
where it came from either by our own legs or by those of the
table, bed or couch on which we lie. But in this return, our
muscles and our joints together play decisive parts. The locomotor system is a kinetic unit.

The Potential Actions of Muscles

We are now in a position to formulate certain tentative
rules governing the use of muscles for the performance of
particular tasks. These rules are based upon our study of myokinematics and myokinetics. Furthermore, they assume that
the principle of muscular economy is observed; and are valid
only insofar as this principle *is* observed. Finally, these rules
have to do with physical events; so, in accordance with the
spirit of modern physics, one of them is of a kind that could
be called "statistical" — in technical language *stochastic* —
for it permits certain variations in the use of muscles for a
particular purpose, not only between different persons but
also in one and the same person at different times.

There are four rules. These are: the Kinematic Rule, two
rules of Kinetic Minimality, and the Statistical Rule. The first
three are stated in terms of *myones*, for these are the ultimate
functional sources of energy and force. The fourth rule is
stated in terms of *muscles*, for they, not their constituent myones, are the only structures in which the operation of the
rule can be observed.

The Kinematic Rule. Only those myones are used that are
necessary as prime movers or synergists for the causation of
the intended angle of swing and/or spin.

The Rule of Minimal Spurt Force. Only as many kinematically suitable myones are used as are both necessary and sufficient for the production of the total spurt force necessary for motion or stabilization.

The Rule of Minimal Shunt Force. Only those kinematically and spurtwise suitable myones are used that are sufficient to secure that the total transarticular force is equal to the total load carried by the bone(s) they act on, together with the centripetal Newtonian force associated with a swing of intended speed.

This rule (if observed!) would determine the set of myones used in stabilization and for varying speeds of motion. It is, therefore, not a corollary (or consequence) of the preceding rule.

The Statistical Rule. Only one muscle can flex the terminal phalanx of a finger or toe. There are no *degrees of muscular freedom* (DMF) in this case. But the second (middle) phalanx can be flexed by the fl. profundus digitorum, which also flexes the third phalanx; by the fl. superficialis digitorum, which flexes this phalanx itself; or by both flexors: in this case there are 3 ways of flexing a phalanx. Now at least one of these three ways must be used if the phalanx is to be flexed; hence we have 2DMF. Finally, each of these two phalanges can be extended by any one of 3 muscles, anatomically anyway: by the ext. communis, by the two interossei (considered as a single muscle) or by the lumbrical; by any two of these; or by the three acting together. There are, then, 7 ways of using the available extensor muscles to extend a terminal or middle phalanx, of which one must be used; so that we have 6 ways of "selecting" the ways that will *not* be used, and this fact is expressed by saying that in this case there are 6 DMF.

These three examples are both necessary and sufficient to establish the following theorem —

Let m be the number of muscles available for performing a particular task of stabilization or motion at a particular joint; then there are ($2^m - 1$) ways in which these muscles can be used (singly, in pairs, in triples ... or all together); and the set of muscles in question has ($2^m - 2$) degrees of (muscular) freedom. This is *The Statistical Rule.*

The rule is so-called because it can be made the basis of electromyographic studies (including existing data) that have been lacking up till now. If the "selection" by the nervous system of one or more muscles of an available set be *purely random*, than the *a priori* probability that *either* a single muscle *or* any particular possible combination of muscles will be used on a single occasion will be precisely $1/(2^m - 1)$. In this quite exact "stochastic probability" we have the foundation of an examination of EMG results with the objective of determining experimental laws that can be used to confirm, modify or deny the other rules we have stated. This book is not the place for developing this statistic, but we can look at a few examples drawn from the chapters that follow this one. Before doing so, however, we would make one relevant remark.*

The fact that, say, two muscles are used for a given task where only one is used on other occasions for the same task does not necessarily conflict with the two rules of Kinetic Minimality; for these rules have to do with myones, and the necessary and sufficient number of myones used for satisfying the rules may be contained in the two muscles together or in one of them only.

Consider pure flexion of an elbow joint. There are 7 muscles crossing this joint on its flexor aspect: these are divisible into a *trio*, composed of biceps, brachialis and brachioradialis; and a *quartet*, composed of the 2 carpal flexors, the pronator teres and the humeral head of flexor digitorum superficialis — we neglect the palmaris longus. There are, therefore (2^7-1), that is, 127 different ways in which the set of seven muscles could be used for elbow flexion. To these 127 ways the trio contributes a total of 2^3, that is, 8. Thus, the stochastic probability that on any *one* occasion elbow flexion would be caused by one or more of the trio *and by no others*; that probability (we say) is 8/127. The probability that the trio would be the only operative set on a second occasion is $(8/127)^2$ — which is 1/252. Finally, the stochastic probability that only one *or* more muscles of the trio would

---

*The probability distribution is that of a "Minimally Incomplete Binomial Type" based on equiprobability of events.

be operative on a fourth occasion approaches 16 in a million; putting it in the language of gamblers (the true tongue of statistics), the odds against any or all members of the trio being used four times in succession are 1,000,000 to 16!

We need go no further. The enormous improbability of one or more muscles of the 'trio' being used four times in succession is based on the hypothesis of random selection of elbow flexors by the nervous system. Electromyography has shown conclusively that it is from within the trio that the musculature of pure elbow flexion is always drawn in fact. The selection of the flexor trio is therefore *prescribed* — to use a term that appears to be justified in this connection.

We now look at the composition of the trio itself. Two of its muscles are of the spurt type, as we know; all of the quartet and the third member of the trio are of the shunt type: so that the use of the trio in pure elbow flexion is statistically very highly significant with respect to the part played by spurt muscles in either stabilization or motion of the forearm. We now look at the muscles within the trio.

As there are 3 muscles, there are in all 7 ways of using them singly or in combination. As there are 2 spurt muscles, the stochastic probability of *at least* one spurt muscle being used in any instance of flexion is 6/7; and that of using only the brachioradialis is 1/7. This means that the stochastic probability of using the brachioradialis alone in 4 instances is just under 1/6000. Thus, the hypothesis of random selection of myones in great part from within the spurt members of the trio appears to be enough to account for the EMG results (see Chapters 8 and Part 3), in most cases anyway.

Enough has been said above, we think, to indicate how a statistical analysis can be made of electromyographic data in any study of the muscles acting on specific joints; and to show the use of the classification into spurt and shunt types in making such an analysis. It is necessary to consider the stochastic ("probability") aspect of myokinesiology because of our ignorance of the precise working of the nervous system in "selecting" the myones for any particular task; and for assessing how far variations *within* individuals are commensurate with differences *between* individuals. And so we pass on to see something of what muscles actually do.

REFERENCES

Basmajian, J.V. (1959) "Spurt" and "shunt" muscles: an electromyographic confirmation. *J. Anat., 93:* 551-553.

Joseph, J. and Nightingale, A. (1957) Electromyography of certain hip muscles. *J. Anat., 91:* 286-294.

MacConaill, M.A. (1946) Some anatomical factors affecting the stabilizing functions of muscles. *Ir. J. Med. Sc., Series vi, 246:* 160-164.

MacConaill, M.A. (1973). The four states of living muscle: a rational nomenclature. *Histology Newsletter.* Anat. Soc. Gr. Brit. & Irel. *2:* 7-8.

Travill, A.A. (1962) Electromyographic study of the extensor apparatus of the forearm. *Anat. Rec., 144:* 373-376.

Main Concepts only

The Actual Action of Muscles

In this chapter we consider the way in which muscles are used in a certain number of instances, with a view to testing the operation of the laws set forth at the end of the preceding chapter. The succeeding chapters greatly enlarge upon the actual action of many specific muscles and groups of muscles. All the evidence is electromyographical, and the reader is referred to Basmajian (1974) for references to the original papers.

Pronation and Supination

Consider the following facts:

The only muscles used for moving or stabilizing the radius at the two radio-ulnar joints are the two pronators, the supinator and the biceps (brachii).

(1) SLOW MOVEMENT. The pronator quadratus is used for pronation, the supinator for supination. There is slight activity in the pronator teres during pronation but the main activity is in quadratus.

(2) QUICK MOVEMENT. Both pronators are active in pronation, the quadratus more so during the passage from semi- to full pronation. Similarly, both supinator and biceps (a supinator) are active, the latter more so during the passage from semi- to full supination. If, however, the elbow be *kept extended* then only the supinator is active.

189

(3) MOVEMENT AGAINST RESISTANCE. Both pronators and both supinators are active in pronation and supination, respectively.

(4) ANTAGONISM. The pronators are *inactive* during supination, the supinators during pronation.

NOTE. The above statements refer to pronation-supination carried out without an accompanying flexion or extension at the elbow.

The Underlying Principles

The above facts illustrate the law of minimal muscle action very clearly. The small pronator quadratus and supinator are used for slow movement, serving as the spurt muscles for the actions they produce. The oblique pull of the supinator is enough to produce a shunt thrust of the radius towards the humerus, but the quite transverse pull of the pronator quadratus does not provide a similar thrust and so the pronator teres is called into play to a minimal degree in order to provide it.

For quick pronation and supination, however, more energy is required and so the pronator teres and biceps are used to assist the pronator quadratus and supinator, respectively. The same remark applies to the use of these "assistant muscles" in pronation-supination against resistance even if the movement be slow.

The fact that quick supination is carried out by the supinator alone when the elbow is extended conforms to the principle of minimal muscle action. The biceps is a flexor as well as a supinator. Were it to be used, then some part of the triceps would have to be used to prevent the flexion that the biceps would bring about. This would entail the use of *three* muscles—a biologically wasteful procedure. Hence the supinator alone is used. The biceps is inhibited in fact; when it is employed in supination against resistance there is usually some accompanying flexion brought about by it.

Finally, it is to be noted that both pronators are uncontracted during supination, both supinators during pronation. Each pair offers passive resistance to the action of the other pair, but only passive resistance—they are mutually *reactive antagonists*, not active antagonists. This, of course, is a further example of minimal muscle action.

Flexion and Extension at the Elbow

Consider the following facts and principles:

There are four muscles actually used for flexing the elbow and two for extending it. Gravity can be used for bringing about either movement, depending upon the rotation of the humerus at the shoulder joint. Since either pronation or supination can be combined with either flexion or extension, there are *six* possible types of motion altogether.

EXTENSION. Only the triceps is involved. This muscle, however, acts only when gravity cannot take its place. The medial (*i.e.*, deep) head is always active, the lateral head slightly so, in unresisted movement. The lateral head is recruited further in resisted extension and the long head acts as a further reserve of power. Here again, then, the law of minimal spurt action is verified.

The brachioradialis is active in *rapid* extension, just as it is in rapid flexion, but is inactive, of course, in slow extension. This is another instance of minimal shunt action, for the shunt effect of this muscle is, of course, independent of the direction of swing of the forearm.

When gravity is used as the prime mover, then the elbow flexors can and do function as active antagonists for regulating the speed of extension. In *slow* extension the brachialis is used for this purpose, yet another example of minimal spurt action.

Flexion of Interphalangeal Joints of Finger

Consider the following facts and principles:

In slow flexion of the two interphalangeal (IP) joints of a finger only the flexor profundus is normally used. Its tendon passes over both joints to its insertion on the distal phalanx and its action on the distal IP joint needs no explanation. Its action on the proximal IP joint is not so obvious, but can be understood by remembering that the carpometacarpal, intercarpal and radiocarpal joints are moved by tendons that pass over them in synovial sheaths to be inserted on metacarpals. The mechanics by which metacarpal swing generates, say, lunate swing at the radiocarpal joint is too complex to be discussed here. But we are perfectly justified in applying what we know by experience about the wrist to the analogous case of the interphalangeal joints.

With a little practice it is possible to flex a proximal IP joint while the distal one is kept extended. In this case only the flexor superficialis is active. Thus IP flexion provides yet another example of the minimal spurt action.

If, however, the IP joints are used for grasping an object forcibly, or if they are flexed rapidly, then both the fl. superficialis and the fl. profundus are used. In the latter case, the superficialis provides an additional shunt force for the proximal IP joint, something unnecessary in slow flexion of this joint.

Stabilization of the Pendent Upper Limb

From EMG studies of the shoulder musculature Basmajian and Bazant (1959) concluded that the whole weight of an unloaded arm is counteracted at the glenohumeral joint by the superior part of its capsule alone, no muscles being required. In this area the coracohumeral ligament can be very strong and would appear to reinforce the action of the joint capsule in preventing the head of the humerus from sliding downwards on the inclined plane formed by the glenoid cavity of the scapula. With moderate or heavy loads the supraspinatus is brought into action to reinforce the original tension in the capsule, and in many of the subjects the muscle was in action even when the only load was that constituted by the upper limb itself. In some instances it was found that the posterior fibres of the deltoid were also called into play, these being more or less parallel to the supraspinatus fibres.

The mechanical problem is shown in fig. 8.1. As the reader knows, the head of the humerus is directed medially towards the glenoid cavity, so that this, and not the shaft of the humerus, is the part of the bone that is moved *within the joint* by external forces. In the pendent position of the limb the humerus articulates with the upper portion of the glenoid cavity. If the diameter of the head taken from its point of contact within the scapula to the greater tuberosity of the humerus (fig. 8.1) be s, and if half this diameter be r, then the weight (W) of the whole upper limb can be presumed to act at right angles to this diameter and half way along it, that is, at a distance r from the contact-point. The weight of the limb will tend to roll the humeral head downwards because it exercises a turning-moment (wr) on the head at the contact-point. If this rolling motion were permitted then the shaft of the humerus would tend to rotate medially, carrying the rest of the limb with it. The prevention of this rolling movement is the essential mechanical problem.

Because only the supraspinatus and/or the upper part of the shoulder capsule are known to be involved, the solution of the problem is clear. It proceeds from two facts: (i) that the upper part of the capsule is actually inserted on to the greater and lesser tuberosities of the humerus and (ii) that the greater part of the supraspinatus is actually inserted into this part of the capsule about half way between the glenoid margin and the greater tuberosity. Hence the supraspinatus can be considered as accessory to the capsule in this connection. If, therefore, a suitable force (F) be applied at the greater tuberosity then it will exercise a moment fs which will balance the moment wr. We would then have

$$fs = f(2r) = wr$$
$$f = w/2$$

That is to say, the force to be exerted would be only half of

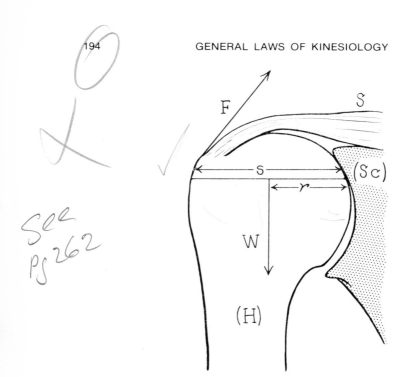

Fig. 8.1. Mechanical scheme (exaggerated) of stabilization of pendent upper limb by supraspinatus (S). The lower part of the head of humerus (H) is in contact with upper part of glenoid cavity of scapula (Sc). The force (F) of a supraspinatus acts upon the line between the point of contact of humerus and scapula and the insertion of the supraspinatus; this line has a half-length *r* and a total length *s*. The weight (W) of the whole upper limb acts through the mid-point of the said line. Further details in text.

the weight of the upper limb, together with any load carried by it.

It would seem that in some cases the tension in the upper part of the capsule is enough to generate this moment; this is an example of a reactive force (Chapter 7). In other cases the supraspinatus must be called in to increase the magnitude of the force (F); and this is always so when a moderate or heavy load is added to that of the limb.

We have here a very striking example of the principle of minimal muscle action, in particular of minimal spurt action.

For example, the upper fibres of infraspinatus and subcapularis could be called into action but this is not done. It should be noted that even when the supraspinatus is not functioning "actively" it is functioning "reactively". Since part of it is inserted on to the joint capsule this cannot be stretched without the muscle being stretched also.

Munro (personal communication) has suggested the mechanical scheme shown in fig. 8.2. He sees the weight of the bone (W) and the supraspinatus force (S) as combining to form a force (F) which presses the humeral head into the glenoid "socket" in all positions of the scapula. This is, we think, true for all positions of the limb except the pendent one. Reference to the figure will show that the resultant of Munro's W and S will act downwards as well as medially; certainly some such force will be required when the humeral

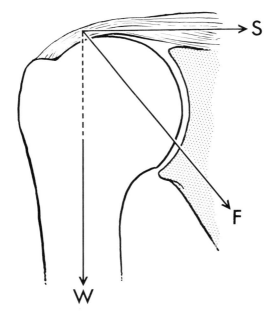

Fig. 8.2. The resolution of forces (F) of W (weight of limb) and S (supraspinatus) tends to force the humeral head into the glenoid fossa.

head moves downwards, as it does during the movement of abduction.

Lastly, it should be remarked that both the capsule and the
supraspinatus muscle have the additional function of preventing the downward slide of the pendent humerus upon the
inclined plane formed by the glenoid cavity (Basmajian and
Bazant, 1959), whether the muscle is "active" or merely "reactive".

Stabilization of the Hip in Standing

When a man stands upright but not in the position of military *Attention*! then the hip joint is nearly but not completely
in the close-packed position. Hence the capsule of the joint
still allows some backward swing of the trunk on the two femoral heads. The joint is in a *metastable* position because of
this. EMG shows that the iliopsoas muscles are the only ones
then active. Clearly, these flexor muscles act to prevent any
backward swing (extension) of the trunk by pulling on the
vertebral column from below—their insertions are now their
functional origins. They and the two recti femoris are the only
muscles capable of counteracting a backward swing of the trunk.
This fact calls for a further analysis of the functional anatomy
of the two pairs of muscles.

When a man is standing upright, both a rectus femoris and
an iliopsoas have their functional origins below the hip joint.
The origin of rectus is far from the joint, its insertion near to
the joint; it is definitely a *spurt* muscle in a standing man. The
origin of iliopsoas is near the joint, its insertion far from it;
it is definitely a *shunt* muscle in a standing man. Why then
is the shunt muscle, iliopsoas, the "muscle of election"?

The answer is this. It is a fact that the quadriceps tendon is
relaxed when a man stands upright. Rectus femoris must act
on the knee as well as on the hip if it contracts. If it were used
to stabilize the hip it would also tense the quadriceps tendon;
therefore it is excluded (or excused!) from action. This leaves
only the iliopsoas as fit for the job: it *must* be used. There is

no need for any other muscle because the trunk is, as it were, in the *antipendent* position dealt with in Chapter 7, and gravity can act as the chief stabilizing factor, allowing of a minimal use of muscle power (see Fujiwara and Basmajian, 1975).

From another point of view it is not unfitting that the iliopsoas set should be used. An iliopsoas has a marked vertically downward pull, so that it acts in the same direction as gravity. It thus assists in generating the pressure that flattens both articulating surfaces, distributing the trunk-weight over a greater area and thus lessening the pressure on each of them. This is an important contribution to stabilization of the joint.

Finally, our analysis has shown, as did our analysis of shoulder stabilization, how important it is to consider all the possible effects of the action of a muscle when we interpret the results of experimental work. To adapt Rudyard Kipling's famous words about England:

> *What do they know of one joint, who only one joint know?*

Stabilization of the Ankle

The ankle joint (crurotalar joint) is one of particular practical importance. No muscles whatever are attached to the talus, nor are any attached to the calcaneus that are relevant in the present connection. Furthermore, the close-packed position of the joint is that of full dorsiflexion, and if we stand upon our feet with the ankle fully dorsiflexed our knees must be flexed. Yet we can stand upright quite comfortably when the tibia is vertical, midway between its positions of full dorsiflexion and full plantar flexion. How can this be?

The answer is found by combining an anatomical investigation of the joint with the results of EMG performed upon subjects standing upright.

Cut away the femur from a knee joint and remove all muscles and tendons from the leg-and-foot portion of the lower limb without, however, destroying the capsules and ligaments of the joints of this portion. We thus obtain an osteoligamentous preparation of what we may call the *pedicrus* for brevity.

Now stand the pedicrus upon a flat table with the crural skeleton (*tibia cum fibula*) vertical. It will remain standing even if the table be hammered gently. If, however, the hammering be violent then the pedicrus will fall.

This experiment shows that the pedicrural skeleton itself is stable rather than unstable when the crural skeleton is vertical. We can assert confidently that it is at least metastable when it is conjoined with the thigh and trunk, if the weight from the trunk be transmitted vertically through the two crura when we stand upright. Each pedicrus will then receive half the weight of the remainder of the body. This weight will tend to flatten the tibial and talar conarticular surfaces by mutual pressure because of the deformability of cartilage, a factor assisting stabilization. We expect to find minimal degree of muscular action, an expectation justified by experiment.

The calf muscles (gastrocnemius, soleus and tibialis posterior) acting from below can prevent forward swing; the tibialis anterior can prevent backward swing. Of these, only the two calf muscles and tibialis anterior are not inserted on the under surface of the arch of the foot; these three muscles, then, are the only ones that *a priori* can act on the ankle alone during standing. Broadly speaking, the calf musculature is either constantly or intermittently active, a finding in accord with the observation that the tibia of the "osteoligamentous pedicrus" tends to fall forwards rather than backwards when the table on which it stands is hammered. The calf musculature here acts in a manner analogous to the iliopsoas at the hip* .

Stabilization of the Foot

There has been a running argument for years upon the question whether the arch of a foot is maintained by muscular ef-

---

*The action of the muscles acting on the ankle will be considered in more detail in Chapter 13.

fort, by ligamentous tension or by a combination of the two, and upon the correlative question of the cause of flat-foot. Those who stressed the rôle of muscles in the affair did so largely on the grounds that ligaments under recurrent, even if not continuous, strain would stretch and so cease to act as efficient "ties" between the anterior and posterior parts of the arch, thus allowing it to collapse. Much of this argument was bedevilled by two errors common to all parties: the notion that collagen fibres were less resistant to tension than muscle and a mistaken notion about the nature of the structure of the foot-skeleton. We shall, therefore, deal with these two errors before considering the results of EMG.

(1) *All skeletal muscles act upon their attachments through collagen fibres.* These fibres at one or both ends of a muscle may not be long enough to be called tendons in textbooks. But they are there nevertheless, and they are tendons in fact. No muscle, therefore, can exert a tension stronger than its collagenous attachments can transmit. From the functional aspect, a muscle could be described as a "ligament of variable length and strength". Its strength increases when it goes into contraction—but so also does the stress it exerts upon its tendons.

When we examine the intrinsic muscles of the sole of the foot (*planta pedis*) we find all grades of muscular structure. We have the highly fleshy abductor hallucis, the semi-muscular, semi-fibrous transverse head of adductor hallucis and the highly fibrous abductor digiti minimi. It is but a short step from the last muscle to, say, the long plantar ligament, a completely collagenous structure.

(2) It was shown in Chapter 5 that only the lateral part of the foot-skeleton is a true arch. The so-called medial arch is a consequence of the fact that the pedal skeleton is a twisted plate, the height of this "arch" depending upon the amount of twist and this depending in turn upon the extent to which the feet are brought together by adduction of the limbs at the hips.

Thus we have not one problem, but two, to solve: that of the maintenance of the lateral arch, which provides the basic curvature of the plantar skeleton, and that of the cause of the pronation (greater twist) of the feet when they are close together.

When we stand with our feet wide apart, then all of the joints between the calcaneus and the metatarsal heads are in close-pack (Chapter 5). Hence the ligaments of this part of the foot-skeleton are the obvious agents for maintaining both the lateral arch and what remains of a medial arch. With these ligaments we can include such highly fibrous muscles as the abductor digiti minimi acting as an additional tie for the lateral arch, and the remaining set of plantar muscles (notably the abductor hallucis), *acting reactively*, even though not contracted, because of their visco-elastic properties—they act as ligaments in fact.

Little more can be said because of a lack of EMG studies comparing muscular activity between near-together and wide-apart feet in standing. Supination of the foot (as we have defined it—untwisting) can be brought about by the action of gravity alone upon wide-apart feet the plantar muscles of which have been "relaxed". What brings about pronation (twisting) in near-together feet is still unknown. Here such muscles as abductor hallucis and the accessorius-complex could well play an active part. Moreover, the principal insertion of tibialis posterior is into the tuberosity of the navicular bone, so that its main action in standing could be to pull this bone backwards against the head of the talus. The corresponding articular surface of the navicular is the anterior part of the *acetabulum pedis* (fig. 5.13) which can be swung slightly forwards and backwards at the hinge shown in the figure. This action of the tibialis posterior would be required in any loose-packed position of the talocalcaneocuboid joint, for example when the feet are close together.

In the study of Basmajian and Stecko (1963) the feet of the (sitting) subject were quite wide apart, so that the arch skeleton was in or near the close-packed position, in which ligamentous support is enough, and the tibialis posterior *inter alia* was inactive accordingly.

Servile Muscles

The reader will have observed that when two or more muscles are capable of carrying out a given action, one of them is always used, either alone or with some other(s). We call such muscles *servile muscles* (*musculi serviles*) from the Latin *servus*, a slave. Examples are the supraspinatus in shoulder stabilization and abduction, the brachialis in elbow-flexion, and the medial (deep) head of triceps brachii in elbow-extension. These are spurt muscles. The shunt muscle, brachioradialis, is also a servile muscle, for it is used in both quick extension and quick flexion of the elbow.

The existence of servile muscles could only be determined after the introduction of EMG. It is of manifest clinical importance, for such muscles are more likely to become fatigued than their more lordly fellows who help them only when they have to. The markedly painful and crippling condition called "frozen shoulder" is caused by the reaction in supraspinatus. It is the shoulder muscle most subject to disturbance, a fact quite understandable from its rôle in support of the pendent upper limb even when the load carried by the limb is considerable. This raises the question of the strength of muscles.

The Strength of Muscles

We define strength by first defining weakness. Nowadays a structure, say a rod, is called weak if it either fractures easily when a stress acts across it or lengthens easily when a tension is applied along it and does not recover its length when the stress is removed, *i.e.*, if it is *ductile but inelastic*. We can talk, then, of *ductile weakness* and hence of *ductile strength;* we are concerned here with these types of weakness and strength alone.

We begin with a simple experiment. Take a fresh muscle belly with a tendon at one end. Clamp the other end of the belly firmly in a vise. Attach the tendon to some device for exerting increasing tension on it. It will be found that the muscle belly will break before the tendon does. The break in the muscle will be found to be due to some of its fibres' having slipped past other fibres.

Now this kind of thing is also found to occur in ductile metals, one row of atoms slipping past a neighbouring row when sufficient tension is applied. The phenomenon is called *dislocation* and is one example of the strain caused by a shearing stress. In fact, the breakage of the muscle is due to a shear strain, the sequence of events being:

(1) Tension along the muscle elongates its fibres.

(2) There comes a point when some fibres can elongate no more.

(3) These fibres either break or are pulled unbroken in the direction of tension past other fibres, thus causing a break in the muscle belly.

This kind of experiment shows that tendon (*i.e.*, collagen) resists tension and shearing stresses better than muscle. This is due in part to the fact that tendons consist of bundles of collagen intertwined like the strands of a rope (fig. 8.3). Muscle fibres, though they may cross one another as in a cruciate muscle, do not coil round one another as do those of a tendon.

Thus the "strength" of a muscle is dependent upon its ability to resist tension due to applied force—that of a weight or of the pull of one or more antagonists. The *internal* breakage of individual muscle fibres is also due to dislocation, this time caused by the string-like molecules of actin and myosin sliding past one another to an over-great extent when the tension forces are too large. It is known from electron microscopy that the actin and myosin molecules do slip past one another in muscular relaxation and slip past one another in the contrary sense during muscular contraction (fig. 8.4). Contraction of a muscle, then, means that a tensile force acts on molecules which are more resistant to "dislocation" than those of a relaxed muscle. The muscle becomes harder, as we know, this hardness being accompanied by a lesser "ductility" than that of a relaxed muscle. This is why muscles in "isometric" contraction can resist external force in the way they do.

From our study of the supraspinatus we must conclude that isometrically contracted muscles are much stronger than might appear at first sight. We can give a numerical estimate. The weight of an adult male's upper limb is about 5670 gm. The supraspinatus weighs about 33 gm. Hence the force balanced by a supraspinatus stabilizing a pendent limb is about 170 times the weight of the muscle *at least*. If a man weighing 140 pounds had the same relative mechanical power as his two supraspinati he could support a weight of about 23 tons by means of a rope and pulley.

The supraspinatus, then, is demonstrably capable of the work it has to do—both stabilizing a pendent limb and as-

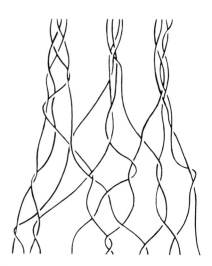

Fig. 8.3. The collagen bundles of a tendon intertwine, here shown teased apart (after Mollier).

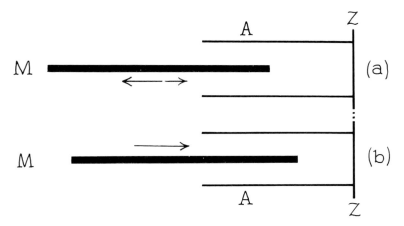

Fig. 8.4. To show the sliding of muscle filaments that occurs when a muscle passes from a relaxed state (a) to the contracted state (b) or *vice-versa*.
The thin actin filaments (A) remain in position; the thick myosin filaments
(M) slide between the actin filaments as shown. ZZ, the Z-line of a muscle
fibre, towards or away from which the myosin filaments slide.

sisting the deltoid in abduction of the arm at the shoulder.
Like all servile muscles it has a very fleshy belly. In the slave
markets of olden days women were chosen largely for their
looks, men for their muscularity. They were forced to be slaves
by those who were even stronger than they and yet would
not work unless compelled to do so by superior authority. We
have our "slave-muscles". The superior authority over the
others is the central nervous system.

The Group Action of Muscles

The term "group action of muscles" signifies the *kinematic*
action of muscles when two or more of them are in action together in producing or preventing movement. It is to be distinguished from the term "mass action of muscles" which has
to do with the total forces generated by these same muscles—
their *kinetic* action.

From the standpoint of group action, muscles are classified

as prime movers, as synergists or as antagonists. A prime mover is the main muscle, sometimes the only muscle, bringing about some action. An antagonist is one that can oppose the action of some prime mover *completely*. A synergist is a muscle that acts as a *partial* antagonist of some prime mover and prevents some unwanted action of the prime mover. When prime movers and their antagonists are in action together then they are referred to conjointly as fixation muscles.

EMG and the accurate analysis of the consequences of motion at joints of more than 1 degree of freedom have greatly modified formerly held views about the group action of muscles. We now know that the use of muscles requiring synergists is avoided as far as possible, for the use of any one such muscle would in fact involve the use of at least one other—a wasteful proceeding. This is why we have servile muscles like the brachialis and the supinator. To use the biceps in slow, simple flexion or supination would require the use of a synergic pronator or extensor, respectively. One of the tasks still to be accomplished by electrokinesiologists (to coin a new word for a very new profession) is the determination of the number of servile muscles we possess.

On the other hand, the phenomenon of conjunct rotation has indicated that synergists act on occasions unthought of in earlier days. A notable example is that of upswing followed by medial deviation of an eyeball, which requires the synergic use of an inferior oblique muscle to prevent the torsion (spin) of the eyeball that would otherwise accompany the medial deviation, the second stage of this diadochal movement.

Sometimes the demands of economy call for the use of two prime movers instead of one! The two carpal flexors and the two carpal extensors are required for their respective purposes. The ulnar flexor and extensor each have some power of ulnar deviation of the hand. It would, then, be wasteful to have a separate adductor carpi for ulnar deviation. Hence the ulnar flexor and extensor are used together for this purpose. They reinforce each other's action as prime movers and are mutual antagonists with respect to carpal flexion and extension. In ulnar deviation, therefore, they could well be described as co-synergists.

Then there is gravity—the "unseen muscle", always used when and insofar as it can do the work required. It is a prime mover in downward movement of a bone, an antagonist in upward movement, and a fixation force in stabilization in the vertical plane, as we have seen. In downward movement it is an accelerating prime mover and requires one or more muscles as decelerating synergists if uniform speed is required. In movement of a bone upwards at a uniform speed it provides part of the deceleration that counters the acceleration of the muscle, and then it is a synergist to the muscular prime mover. It is to be noted that the spurt muscles are the anti-gravity muscles both for stabilization and for movement.

Finally, there are the shunt muscles. These act at high speeds of joint movement to prevent the spurt musculature from straining or even dislocating the joint—both unwanted effects of the prime movers! Hence we must class shunt muscles as synergists.

We have already seen that antagonists come into action against prime movers less frequently than used to be thought. If, however, two bones in a horizontal position are stabilized at their common joint, then the prime movers and their antagonists act together.

The importance of the classification implied by "group action" is that synergy can occur even when *voluntary* use of the prime movers is impossible. It is controlled by the extrapyramidal part of the central nervous system, particularly by the cerebellum. Disease of the subcortical nervous system can, therefore, lead to asynergic use of muscles. This, however, is outside the scope of our book.

REFERENCES

Basmajian, J.V. (1974). *Muscles Alive: Their Functions Revealed by Electromyography,* 3rd Ed., Williams & Wilkins Co., Baltimore.

Basmajian, J.V. and Bazant, F.J. (1959). Factors preventing downward dislocation of the adducted shoulder joint: an electromyographic and morphological study. *J. Bone and Joint Surg. 41A:* 1182-1186.

Basmajian, J.V. and Stecko, G. (1963). The role of muscles in arch support of the foot. *J. Bone and Joint Surg. 45A:* 1184-1190.

Fujiwara, M. and Basmajian, J.V. (1975). Electromyographic study of two-joint muscles. *Am. J. Phys. Med., 54:* 234-242.

MacConaill, M.A. (1949). The movements of bones and joints. II. Function of musculature. *J. Bone and Joint Surg., 31B:* 100-104.

MacConaill, M.A. (1966). The geometry and algebra of articular kinematics. *Bio-Med. Eng., 1:*205-212.

Part Three
SPECIAL KINESIOLOGY

NINE

Vertebral Column

General understanding of the dynamic function of the human back remains woefully inadequate. A host of superstitions and doubtful ideas cluster around this vital area. Indeed, their number surpasses the numerous joints and muscles of the vertebral column.

More than in any other part of the body, posture of the spine has become almost synonymous with general posture. The doctrines of ideal posture, which often take on an evangelic tone, are almost always concerned with the vertebral column. So long as human backs hurt or become deformed, the controversies will live on. In this chapter we shall limit ourselves to examining the basis of vertebral posture and movement. In good conscience we cannot, and we will not, proclaim new theories of ideal posture. On the other hand, the following paragraphs might give little if any comfort to those who have strong views on this subject.

There is no question that the human spine is unique in many ways. Nevertheless, man shares with all vertebrates the common heritage of the several obvious functions served by the vertebral column. These include *protection*—not only of the neural axis or spinal cord but also of the thoracic and abdominal organs, axial *support* of the trunk, and a resilient *mobility* which makes locomotion possible in a multitude of wonderful ways ranging from slithering to flying.

In man, the upright posture has gained the reputation of

being a mixed blessing. Many persons slip all too easily into making the assumption—completely unproved—that man is more heir to a wide range of spinal disabilities than are related quadrupeds. We would reject rather than accept without skepticism the general view put so eloquently by Steindler (1955):

The phylogenetic development of the upright position and the independent functions of the upper extremity have greatly increased the dynamic demands made on the spinal column. In complying with all intricate require-ments, the human spine has developed into a complicated and delicate mechanical unit, the construction of which has placed high demands upon nature's ingenuity.

In such statements there undoubtedly live some elemental truths. But the general statement is mystical rather than scientific and therefore must not form the premise upon which we shall base our discussion. We do not reject phylog-eny; indeed, as anatomists, we have the greatest respect for its lessons. Our *caveat* is against facile acceptance of modern man's evolution when it is used to explain either the normal function of his back or its disabilities. In particular we reject the widespread notion that man's back is the bungled end-result of his renouncing the trees. Cause or effect, the spinal column is a mechanism with potentiality that far exceeds its defects. We shall explore these mechanisms without prejudice other than scientifically sound physics and experimentally verified theory.

In all their many forms, posture and locomotion constantly involve the vertebral column. Thus our concern is with all factors that bear upon both the maintenance of its rigidity in different postures and the motor power that moves the spinal column in whole or in part. The static function of the spine is not simply that of a firm wand. Neither is it as unstable as one might think on viewing its many small parts. We shall now examine the principles underlying the stability of the column and later examine its mobility.

Stability of the Vertebral Column

Curvatures

The history of erect posture in the individual is linked with the   development of the anteroposterior curves of the spine characteristic of the adult. The newborn has only two curves, both concave forward (fig. 9.1). On increasingly assuming first the "heads-up" and then the seated and standing postures, he acquires secondary curves in the neck and lumbar region which allow a vertical and effort-less balance along the sinuous column and through the centre of gravity. In everyday functions, these compensa-

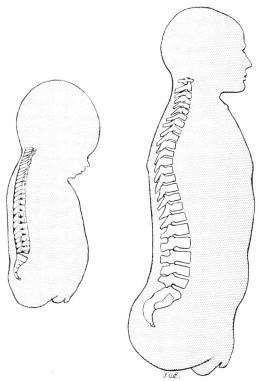

Fig. 9.1. Curves of newborn and adult vertebral columns compared.

tory curves are often flattened or even reversed quite readily. Then the shift of the centre of gravity requires new muscular contractions that provide dynamic guy-wires to prevent overbalancing of the trunk.

While standing erect, most human subjects require very slight activity and sometimes only intermittent reflex activity of the intrinsic muscles of the back. Various investigators have shown by electromyography that during forward flexion there is marked activity until flexion is extreme, at which time the ligamentous structures assume the load and the muscles become silent (figs. 9.2, 9.3). In the extreme-flexed position of the back, the erector spinae remains relaxed in the initial stages of heavy weight-lifting. This observation appears to confirm strongly the dangers of overloading the vertebral ligaments and joints when lifting "with the back" rather than with the leverage and muscular force of the lower limb.

The problems of static posture revolve around the truism that the balance or equilibrium of the human body or its articulated parts depends on a fine neutralization of the forces of gravity by internal counterforces. These counterforces may be supplied most simply both internally and externally by a supporting horizontal surface or series of horizontal surfaces that are wholly inert. The easiest posture in which a human spine can achieve equilibrium with gravity with little if any expenditure of energy is the recumbent one. This is our normal posture for the first year or so of our lives and for about half of our lives thereafter. When we lie down, we bring the centre of gravity of the entire body as well as any or all of its parts closest to a supporting antigravitational surface.

Centre of Gravity

The weight-centre of the whole body is situated at the level of the second sacral vertebra. (On the surface of the body this vertebra is at the level of the posterior superior iliac spines.)

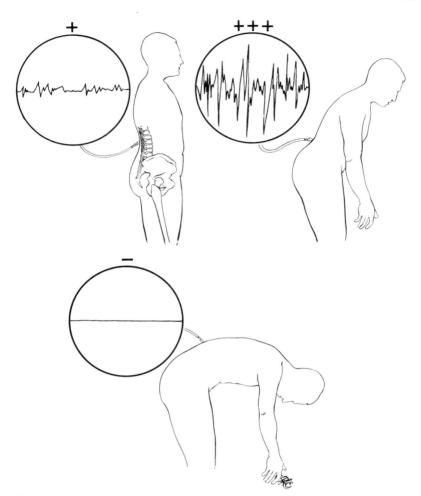

Fig. 9.2. Electromyographic activity in the erector spinae compared in different positions.

In the coronal plane the exact point lies 5 cm. or less behind the line joining the hip joints, and of course it is in the mid-line. To maintain an equilibrium in a standing position with the least expenditure of internal energy, a vertical line dropped from the centre of gravity should fall downward

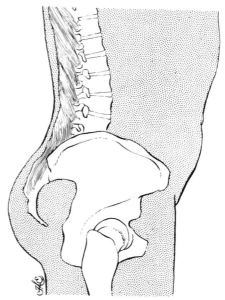

Fig. 9.3. Multifidus as a dynamic posterior "ligament" of the lumbar region.

through an *inert* supporting column of bones and their uniting ligaments.

The idealized normal erect posture is one in which the line of gravity drops in the midline between the following bilateral points: (1) the mastoid processes, (2) a point just in front of the shoulder joints, (3) the hip joints (or just behind), (4) a point just in front of the centre of the knee joints and (5) a point just in front of the ankle joints (fig. 9.4). Muscular activity is called upon only to approximate this posture or, if the body is pulled out of the line of gravity, to bring it back into line. Man has an economical antigravity mechanism once the upright posture is attained; thus his expenditure of muscular energy while standing erect is actually extremely economical (fig. 9.2).

In man, the column of bones that carries the weight to the hip bone and thence to the ground constitutes a series of

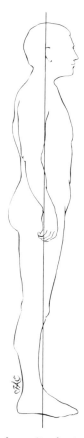

Fig. 9.4. The line of gravity during relaxed standing.

links. Ideally, these should be so stacked that the line of gravity passes directly through the centre of each joint between the links, *i.e.* the intervertebral discs and vertebral bodies. But this ideal is only closely approached—never completely achieved—and then only momentarily. Thus ligaments (constantly) and muscles (intermittently) play vital compensatory roles.

As Steindler (1955) showed, a completely passive equilibrium is impossible because the centres of gravity of the links and the movement-centres of the joints between them cannot all be brought to coincide perfectly with the common line of gravity. In spite of this, we believe that Steindler and many others have greatly exaggerated the amount of effort required to maintain the upright posture. The fatigue of standing in the back (and in the lower limbs) is emphatically not due to muscular fatigue, and generally, the muscular activity in standing is slight or moderate (Donisch and Basmajian, 1972).

Ligamentous factors and the part played by articular processes are discussed below (p. 219).

Movements of Vertebral Column

The vertebral column, the great stabilizer of the trunk, also embodies mobility. However, this mobility is limited by the various ligaments, articular facets, spinous processes, intervertebral discs and other indirect factors. Although the total range of movement of the spine is wide, movement between adjacent vertebrae is quite limited, except for the first two cervical vertebrae (the atlas and axis). Movements

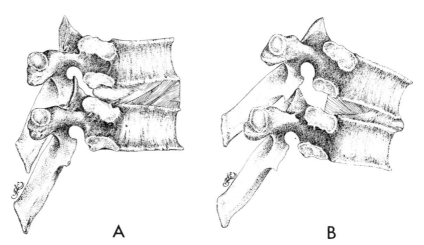

A   B

Fig. 9.5. Hyperextension (A) and flexion (B) of the spinal column cause tension or compression in different parts of an intervertebral disc.

between vertebrae take place by compression in one part and traction in another part of the intervetebral disc (fig. 9.5) and by gliding of the opposed articular processes upon each other (fig. 9.6).

Flexion is bending forward of the trunk. Extension is the opposite movement; when carried backward beyond the erect posture, it is usually called hyperextension. Bending sideways is lateral flexion. Rotation on a vertical axis is called either rotation or torsion.

INTERVERTEBRAL DISCS. In the cervical region the discs are relatively large in comparison with the sizes of the bodies. Flexion is easy in all directions and the articular facets allow free flexion, extension, lateral flexion (especially when accompanied by rotation) and rotation.

The thoracic intervertebral discs are relatively thin. Along with other factors, this limits free movements of the thoracic area. Flexion and extension are limited by the splinting and buttressing effects of the thoracic cage, by the configuration

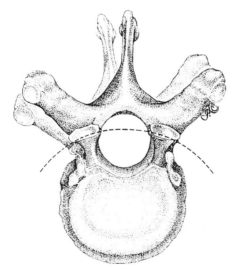

Fig. 9.6. Rotation of thoracic vertebrae is allowed by the configuration of the articular processes.

of the articular facets and by the close overlapping of the spines.

The large lumbar intervertebral discs are very thick and allow free flexion, extension and lateral flexion. The lumbar region is the pivot for most general movements of the trunk, and movements of the lumbar area are most free in the lower lumbar segments. Nevertheless, rotation is limited in the lumbar region by the orientation of the articular facets which tend to intersect the line of rotation.

The total amount of flexion and of rotation in the spine is often overestimated by the unwary. One must not be deceived by the free movements in the hip joint and in the atlanto-occipital joint that occur automatically when a subject is asked to rotate his trunk.

Generally in the cervical and thoracic regions extension is quite free, and modest hyperextension is possible. In the lumbar region and in the lower one or two thoracic segments, hyperextension is sometimes dramatic, as exemplified by professional contortionists. Some slight lateral flexion is possible at all levels, and is most marked at the thoracolumbar junction.

Rotation and lateral flexion are most free in the upper parts of the spine and less free as we pass downward, being almost wholly prevented in the lumbar region by the processes. Lateral flexion and rotation of the spine are almost inseparable. If a flexible rod is bent first in one plane and then, while it is in this bent position, it is bent again in a plane at right angles to the first, it always rotates on its longitudinal axis at the same time (fig. 9.7). This is really an example of consequential conjunct rotation (Chapter 4). As pointed out by Rasch and Burke (1963), when a subject bends forward, exaggerating a condition already present in the thoracic region, a tension is put on the ligaments at the rear (ligamenta flava and interspinous ligaments) that makes them resist lateral flexion more than usual, while the weight, bearing

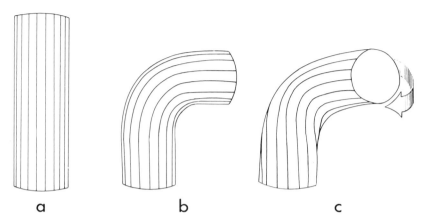

Fig. 9.7. Flexing a rod in two planes produces a twist (see text).

down on the front edges of the bodies, aids in the lateral bend-ing. The result is that the bodies of the vertebrae go farther away from the vertical than do the spinous processes during lateral flexion. The concave side of the normal curve, being under pressure, turns to a convex side of the lateral curve.

It follows that in the thoracic region a lateral bend rotates the spinous processes to the concave side and in the lumbar region to the convex side (fig. 9.8). The rotation which ac-companies lateral flexion is a passive mechanical phenomenon and does not require active contraction of rotator muscles. Furthermore, it is a local effect which seldom achieves suffi-cient magnitude to produce an externally-visible turning of the shoulders in relation to the hips.

When lateral flexion of the trunk is performed, the maxi-mum movement occurs in the lumbar region and at the thoracolumbar junction. There is only slight involvement of the lower thoracic spine. The torsion occurs in the same part of the spine and consists in a turning of the vertebral bodies toward the side of the lateral flexion.

If the lateral flexion is performed from a position of hyper-extension and the hyperextension is maintained, the lateral

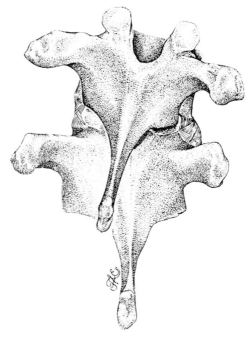

Fig. 9.8. A lateral flexion of a thoracic vertebra rotates its spinous process to the convex side.

flexion occurs almost entirely below the eleventh thoracic vertebra. The position of hyperextension seems to "lock" the thoracic part of the column, bringing it into close-pack.

If the lateral flexion is performed from a position of forward flexion, the movement occurs higher in the spine than ordinarily. The greatest bending occurs at the level of the eighth thoracic vertebra. Now the torsion of the vertebrae reverses itself. In bending to the right while in a flexed position the vertebral bodies turn to the left, and the spinous processes to the right.

Muscular Influences

The erector spinae becomes quite active during forward flexion of the vertebral column. Therefore, one main function is this controlled "paying out", which here is as important as the obvious function of extension (fig. 9.2).

In very rapid flexion, little or no activity is required of erector spinae and none appears. As the slowly flexing trunk is lowered, the activity in erector spinae increases apace and then decreases to quiescence when full flexion is reached. If an attempt is then made to force flexion further, silence continues to prevail in the erector. In full flexion, then, the weight of the torso is borne by the posterior ligaments and fasciae—the posterior common ligament, the ligamentum flavum, the interspinous ligaments and the thick dorsal aponeurosis. The erector spinae again comes into action when the trunk is raised once more to the erect position.

The position of full flexion while seated (usually considered by school teachers as a "bad" posture) is maintained comfortably for long periods and during this time erector spinae remains relaxed. As Floyd and Silver (1950) pointed out, "certain people experience backache if they sit in the fully flexed position for a sufficient time—e.g., patients sitting in bed with only the thoracic part of the vertebral column supported, motor-car drivers, etc." Apparently a reflex inhibitory mechanism explains the complete relaxation of erector spinae in full flexion.

Most subjects standing in a relaxed erect posture show a low level of activity in the erector spinae. Small adjustments of the position of the head, shoulders or hands can abolish the activity of the muscle, *i.e.*, an equilibrium or balance is achieved. From the easy upright posture, extension or hyperextension of the trunk is initiated, as a rule, by a short burst of activity.

While a subject is standing upright, flexion of the trunk to one side is accompanied by activity of the erector spinae of the opposite side, *i.e.*, the muscle is not a prime mover, but an "antagonist". However, if the back is already arched in extension (hyperextension), not even this sort of activity occurs.

Erectores spinae contract (apparently vigorously) during coughing and straining. This occurs even in the midst of their normal silence whether the subject is erect or "full-flexed".

During the performance of various trunk movements, different layers and parts of the spinal musculature—iliocostalis in the thoracic and lumbar parts, longissimus, rotatores and multifidus muscles—show patterns of activity that clearly have two functions. Sometimes they initiate movement and at other times they stabilize the trunk. Almost all the movements recruit all the muscles of the back in a variety of patterns, although the predominance of certain muscles is also obvious (Morris et al., 1962).

In compound movements, when subjects are not trying to relax, there is constantly more activity than when the movement is carried out deliberately and with conscious effort to avoid unnecessary activity of muscles. Complete relaxation and lower levels of contraction are the "ideal" rather than the rule for normal bending movements. Muscles that might be expected to return the spine to the vertical position often remain quiet; this suggests that such factors as ligaments and passive muscle elasticity play an important rôle.

Longissimus

During easy standing, longissimus is slightly to moderately active; it can be relaxed by gentle ("relaxed") extension of the spine. During forced full extension, flexion, lateral flexion and rotation in different positions of the trunk, it is almost always prominently active.

Iliocostalis

A position of complete silence is easily found for this muscle in the erect position, but with slight forward swaying activity is instantly recruited. Forward flexion and rotation in the flexed position bring out its strongest contractions, but it is also fairly active in most movements of the spine.

Multifidus and Rotatores

Multifidus and rotatores have rather similar but not identical activities. With movements in the sagittal plane, they are active. They are also active in contralateral movements in the lumbar region. Paradoxically, rotary movements recruit the deep thoracic rotatores and multifidus muscles almost symmetrically (Donisch and Basmajian, 1972).

Vigorous Movements

Semispinalis capitis and cervicis apparently help to support the head by continuous activity during upright posture (Pauly, 1966). In almost all vigorous exercises performed from the orthograde position, the most active muscle is spinalis; next in order is longissimus, and least is iliocostalis lumborum. Nevertheless all three muscles and the main mass of erector spinae act powerfully during strong arching of the back in the prone posture. During push-ups, there is considerable individual variation, but typically, the lower back muscles remain relaxed.

Simple side-bending exercises of the trunk do not recruit erector spinae so long as there is no concomitant backward or forward bending. This clearly refutes earlier opinions of authors who had ignored movements in the ventro-dorsal plane that do involve erector spinae.

During walking on the level, two periods of activity are found in the sacrospinalis: one during the swinging and one during the supporting phase. The bilateral activity prevents imbalance of the whole body and also rotation and lateral flexion of the trunk.

REFERENCES

Donisch, E.W. and Basmajian, J.V. (1972). Electromyography of deep muscles of the back in man. *Am. J. Anat.*, *133*: 25-36.
Floyd, W.F. and Silver, P.H.S. (1950). Electromyographic study of patterns of activity of the anterior abdominal wall muscles in man. *J. Anat.*, *84*: 132-145.

Morris, J.M., Benner, F. and Lucas, D.B. (1962). An electromyographic study of the intrinsic muscles of the back in man. *J. Anat., 96:* 509-520.

Pauly, J.E. (1966). An electromyographic analysis of certain movements and exercises. I. Some deep muscles of the back. *Anat. Rec., 155:* 223-234.

Rasch, P.J. and Burke, R.K. (1963). *Kinesiology and Applied Anatomy: The Science of Human Movement,* 2nd Ed., Lea & Febiger, Philadelphia.

Steindler, A. (1955). *Kinesiology of the Human Body under Normal and Pathological Conditions,* Charles C Thomas, Springfield, Ill.

TEN

Thoraco-Abdominal Wall

In this chapter we shall consider the mechanisms of movement of the thoracic cage, diaphragm and abdominal wall (especially for breathing), activities of the thorax and abdomen associated with the general posture and mobility of the trunk, and activities concerned with expulsion or retention of the hollow viscera.

Thoracic Cage

The act of inspiration increases the capacity of the thoracic cage in the three principal directions. The transverse diameter is increased by the ribs' swinging outward (fig. 10.1); the antero-posterior diameter is increased by the sternal body's swinging forward, hinge-like, at the sternal angle between it and the relatively stable manubrium sterni (fig. 10.2); the vertical diameter is increased by the piston-like descent and flattening of the dome of the diaphragm. In ordinary quiet breathing, the last factor may well be the most significant. In any case, inspiration is almost wholly an active phenomenon produced by muscular contraction, while the motive power of expiration is passive, depending on the elastic recoil of both the lung and the thoracic wall.

Possible Movements of Ribs

Although it is fair to surmise that each rib has its own pattern of movements, certain generalizations can be made:

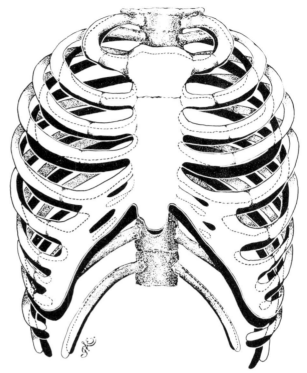

Fig. 10.1. Movements of the rib that increase the transverse diameter of the thorax.

The *first ribs* are so firmly united to the manubrium sterni by their costal cartilages that with it they form a firm horse-shoe-shaped arch which moves only as a unit (fig. 10.3). This movement occurs at the heads of these ribs and essentially is a simple elevation of the manubrium upward and forward.

The *vertebrosternal ribs* (2–7) not only rise upward and forward at their anterior ends, but their lateral (or midshaft) portions will rise in the manner of a bucket-handle (fig. 10.4). Here the axis would seem to be an imaginary line joining the head of a rib to the joint between its costal cartilage and the side of the sternum.

The *next three ribs* (8–10) combine the elevation of their

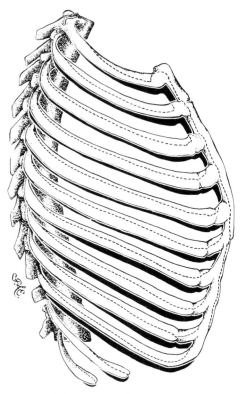

Fig. 10.2. Movements of the ribs and sternum that increase the antero-posterior diameter of the thorax.

anterior ends with a caliper-like opening. The joints of the costal tubercles with the transverse processes of the vertebrae bear witness to this: they are flat and are placed superiorly where the tubercle can slide back and forth with the movement fulcrum at the costal head (fig. 10.5).

The *floating ribs* (11 and 12), as their name implies, are very mobile. The loose joint at their heads and the lack of any union with the transverse processes leave them subject to pushes and pulls in any direction, hinging on the head.

Fick (1911) showed that the ribs also change their shapes, being longer in inspiration as a result of straightening of their

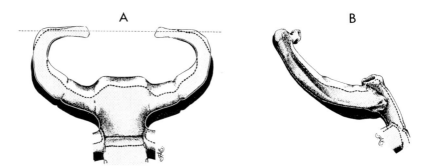

Fig. 10.3. The first ribs and manubrium move upward and forward as a unit.

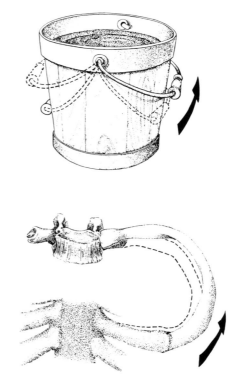

Fig. 10.4. The bucket-handle movement of the typical (vertebrosternal) ribs.

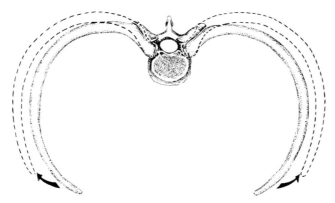

Fig. 10.5. The caliper-like movements of the lowest ribs.

angles. Steindler (1955) stated that the costochondral angles are smallest in forced expiration, somewhat wider at rest and much straightened out during maximum inspiration (fig. 10.6).

Sternal Movements

As a consequence of all the movements of the upper ten ribs, the sternum moves in three ways, all of which blend together. The anteroposterior hinge-like movement of the body (at the sternal angle of Louis) combines with a rise of the manubrium anteroposteriorly as well as the rise of the entire sternum as a unit (fig. 10.2). These movements result in the following average displacements (Strasser, 1913):

Upper border of sternum: movement up—14–17 mm.
                           movement forward—9–12 mm.
Lower end of sternum: movement up—11–12 mm.
                           movement forward—21–24 mm.

Actual Thoracic Movements and Muscular Action during Respiration

Accumulating evidence now suggests that in ordinary quiet respiration thoracic mobility is minimal in normal persons, the diaphragm being the main muscle of respiration. At birth the

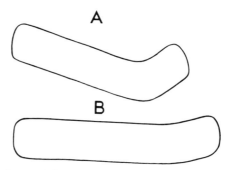

Fig. 10.6. The ribs straighten at the costochondral junctions at maximum inspiration (B).

ribs are horizontal and are in a position of full inspiration; thus in early life the diaphragm is exclusively the respiratory muscle. By the end of the second year the ribs have acquired their shape and thoracic respiration becomes significant. In deep breathing, costal movement is extensive.

The usual concept of normal quiet breathing has been that the scalenes anchor or fix the first rib while the external intercostals elevate the remaining ribs towards the first—this in spite of radiographs showing no approximation of the ribs. Various investigators, particularly Jones, Beargie and Pauly (1953) and Raper *et al.* (1966), showed that both sets of intercostals in man are slightly active *constantly* during quiet breathing and show no rhythmic increase and decrease. In contrast with this, the scalenes show a rhythmic increase during inspiration (figs. 10.7, 10.8).

With forced inspiration, the scalenes, the sternomastoid and the internal and external intercostals show marked activity. In contrast, with forced expiration, the scalenes are quiescent while the intercostals remain active. Therefore, the scalenes are fundamental muscles of inspiration. The intercostal muscles supply the tension necessary "to keep the ribs at a constant distance from each other while the chest is expanded from above and contracted from below" (Jones *et al.*, 1953).

A

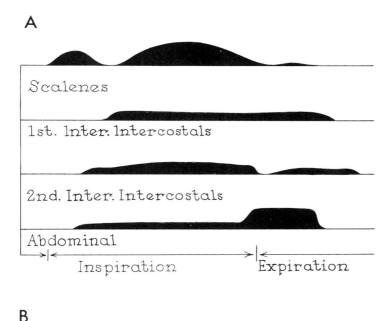

B

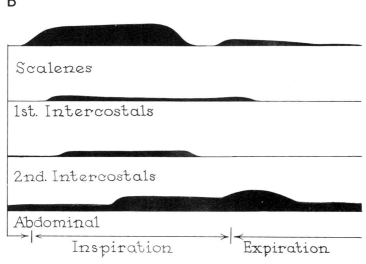

Fig. 10.7. Schematic representation of EMG activity during respiration (based on research reports of several authors, chiefly Jones, Beargie and Pauly, 1953).

A

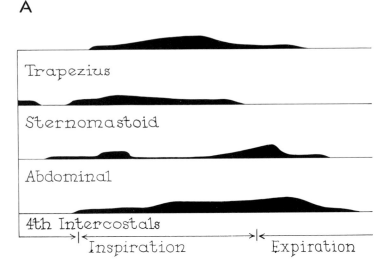

B

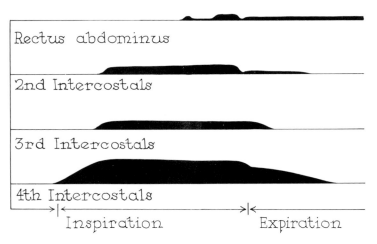

Fig. 10.8. Schematic representation of EMG activity during respiration (based on research reports of several authors, chiefly Jones, Beargie and Pauly, 1953).

Passive membranes between the ribs instead of muscles would be inadequate because they would be sucked in and blown out during respiration, and they would not provide the constant fine control of the rib positions. Moreover, the intercostals function in flexion of the trunk (as in sitting up from the supine position) and so are postural muscles as well. Perhaps the intercostal muscles are used in nonrespiratory activity more than in ordinary respiration.

The main rôle in human respiration is performed by the diaphragm, while the intercostals are necessary for markedly increasing the intrathoracic pressure. A person with paralyzed intercostals has a sharp reduction of sucking and blowing power with comparatively much less embarrassment of quiet respiration (Hoover, 1922).

There are two functionally distinct layers of intercostal muscle everywhere except anteriorly in the interchondral region and posteriorly in the areas medial to the costal angles (Taylor, 1960). Where there are two functional layers, the superficial one (external intercostal) may act only during inspiration and the deeper (internal intercostal) during expiration. In quiet breathing, whatever activity occurs is limited to the parasternal region during inspiration—here there is only one functional layer and it is exclusively internal intercostal. During expiration, in quiet breathing, activity is limited to the lower lateral part of the thoracic cage, coming from the internal intercostals. Apparently there is no external intercostal activity whatsoever in quiet breathing. The transversus thoracis is purely expiratory in function—including its parts known as sternocostalis, intercostales intimi and subcostalis.

More vigorous respiratory effort brings the layers of muscular activity into reciprocal action all over the chest wall. Now the external layer is entirely inspiratory and the internal layer expiratory.

Diaphragmatic Respiration

As indicated earlier, the main respiratory muscle in man is the diaphragm. Although a common belief is that it is a tripartite organ (consisting of the right and left costal parts and the crura forming one part), the diaphragm functions as a unit during inspiration (Boyd and Basmajian, 1963). Studies of diaphragmatic activity in many species including man show that there is little if any activity during expiration.

Phases of Respiration

Quiet respiration includes not only the two simple opposite phases of inspiration and expiration but also a static phase before each—pre-inspiration and pre-expiration. In duration, they are much shorter than the air-moving phases; nonetheless, the static phases make up an appreciable part of the respiratory cycle and are termed inspiratory and expiratory "pauses" in man.

PRE-INSPIRATION. Diaphragmatic activity is slight in this brief phase (fig. 10.9). The onset of contraction in man occurs as much as one-fourth of a second before the onset of inspiration.

INSPIRATION is an increase in the volume of the thorax with an actual inward flow of air. The diaphragm contracts and increases the cavity in a caudad direction and perhaps in the ventrodorsal and lateral directions as well. The activity of the diaphragm increases at the onset of inspiration, and as this phase proceeds, new units are added or "recruited" so that the inspiratory effect gains force as it proceeds. As inspiration continues, the individual motor units in the diaphragm accelerate in rate, resulting in a progressive increment in the strength of contraction.

The peak of the inspiratory motor unit activity terminates

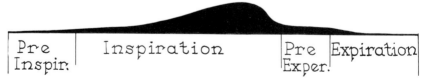

Fig. 10.9. Schematic representation of EMG activity in the diaphragm during various phases of respiration.

before the end of inspiration. In most instances, the peak is followed by a rapid decline—and in some instances by a very sharp drop to the base line, where varying degrees of activity continue to the end of the fourth quarter of the inspiration. Activity never stops at the end of inspiration in man, but electromyographic silence may follow inspiration in other species, *e.g.*, rabbits.

PRE-EXPIRATION is a regular precursor of expiration. During passive expiration, activity always continues from inspiration into expiration.

EXPIRATION, the last phase in the respiratory cycle, consists of a decrease in the volume of the thorax with air moving outward. One way that this might be accomplished is by the contraction of the abdominal muscles, forcing the diaphragm up into the thorax. During quiet breathing, however, expiration is generally regarded as essentially passive. Nonetheless, some activity in the diaphragm has been recorded during expiration. In almost every instance, the (slight) activity lasts for a longer period of time than the greater activity that occurs in inspiration. In man, the activity continues through as much as 98% of expiration (Murphy *et al.*, 1959).

During forced expiration there is no activity originating in the human diaphragm, although activity occasionally carries over from deep inspiration. One possible reason why activity carries into or continues throughout expiration in quiet breathing is that activity in the diaphragm during passive expiration is a braking action to oppose the normal elastic recoil of the lungs. In effect, it is not a true expiratory effort. The anatomical structure of the diaphragm supports this view, because all of its fibres are arranged in radiating fasciculi inserting into the central tendon. Shortening of the fibres can only cause a flattening of the dome and so actually resist the production of an expiratory force. Furthermore, no electrical activity occurs during *forced* expiration.

The rate of airflow at the onset of expiration does not rise rapidly to a maximum (as would be expected if the muscles of inspiration relaxed immediately), indicating that during the early part of expiration the muscles of inspiration decrease their force of contraction only gradually (Campbell, 1958). Measurements of the work of breathing based on pressure-volume diagrams suggest that the muscles of inspiration may exert considerable force in opposing the elastic recoil of the lungs during expiration. This tends to confirm that the slight activity recorded from the diaphragm during expiration is a braking action to oppose the normal elastic recoil of the lungs.

Abdominal Wall

When a person lies supine and resting, the abdominal muscles remain completely relaxed. With the "head raising" movement used commonly as an exercise for strengthening abdominal muscles, the recti are powerfully active while at first the external oblique and the lower part of internal oblique are only slightly active. Even with increased effort they become only moderately active. Only the rectus is benefited maximally by the head-raising exercise, but the bilateral leg-raising exercise brings all the abdominal musculature into activity to steady the pelvis. One-sided leg-raising is much less effective, calling upon activity predominantly on the same side of the abdomen.

In the relaxed standing position, all but the lower part of the internal oblique is inactive. Internal oblique apparently is on constant guard over the inguinal region (see below).

When a person (whether recumbent or erect) strains or "bears down" with the breath held, the external obliques and internal obliques (lower parts) contract to a degree that is directly related to the effort, but rectus abdominis, in contrast, remains very quiet.

There is no inspiratory or expiratory activity in the abdominal muscles during quiet breathing. With forced expiration, with coughing and with singing, the pattern is similar to that in straining, i.e., marked activity in the obliques and none in the rectus. The rectus sheath is very important in protecting the abdominal area occupied by the rectus during all these physiological functions which are *not* accompanied by contraction of the rectus. The apparent hardening of the recti on straining, coughing, etc. is usually only a passive bulging of the muscles and their sheaths.

Movements of the trunk performed without resistance in either the sitting or the standing posture leave the obliques and recti inactive. However, lateral bending of the trunk does produce activity in the more posterolateral fibres of external oblique. Inclining the trunk backwards gives activity in all the muscles, but forward bending is unaccompanied by activity.

During forced trunk-twisting exercises the internal oblique of the side to which the twisting occurs is greatly active, while both external obliques show some slight activity and the recti none at all (unless the subject violently flexes the trunk simultaneously).

The upper and lower parts of the rectus abdominis vary in response to different movements (Flint, 1965). Most of the activity in the recti during trunk flexion from the supine position occurs during the first half of the movement. Trunk raising elicits more activity than trunk lowering.

Postural Rôle of Abdominal Muscles

The rectus abdominis does not draw a resistant spine forwards; gravity does this. Only in full-flexion does rectus show activity, apparently in an effort to force the trunk further downwards against resistance. In hyperextension (at the other end of the range of motion) the rectus abdominis shows activity while being stretched; this apparently steadies the torso. The abdominal muscles are inactive during walking on the level (Sheffield, 1962).

Morris, Lucas and Bresler (1961) and Bearn (1961) have stressed the importance of the abdominal muscles in the development of positive pressure in the abdomen. This is said to be an important adjunct to the vertebral column in stabilizing the trunk.

Control of Inguinal Canal

In the consideration of the abdominal wall posture, we must consider in particular the lower part of region of threatening hernia. Here the inguinal canal tunnels throught the muscular layers of the abdominal wall and so provides a weak spot. Through this area excessive intra-abdominal pressures (particularly while the person is standing) may force a hernia. Since, in the male, the opening transmits the ductus (or vas) deferens, it must be protected without, however, causing complete occlusion. This delicate, but dynamic, function is performed by the internal oblique and transversus abdominis—in particular by their lowest fibres, which arise from the inguinal ligament. These fibres arch over the inguinal canal and insert medially on the pubic bone. They are in constant contraction during standing, and straining and coughing require increased activity in the muscular protection of the canal.

Respiratory Rôle of Abdominal Muscles

There is no activity in the external oblique and rectus abdominis of supine normal subjects breathing quietly. With maximal voluntary expiration these muscles contract as they also do towards the end of maximal voluntary inspiration (figs. 10.7, 10.8). Yet they do not contract under the latter condition when the breathing is increased by imposing asphyxia. In contrast, the activity in maximal expiration increases further when the volume of breathing is increased by asphyxia.

Contracting of the abdominal muscles to aid expiration occurs only in severe cases of greatly increased pulmonary ventilation under stress. In any case, they do not initiate the expiratory phase but rather help to complete it quickly.

In summary, the abdominal muscles are the most important and the only indisputable muscles of expiration in man. The obliques and transversus are much more important than the rectus abdominis. Vigorous contraction occurs in all voluntary expiratory manoeuvres (such as coughing, straining, vomiting, etc.) The abdominal muscles (almost exclusively the obliques) contract at the end of maximum inspiration to help limit its depth, but, in normal persons, they do not contract in hyperpneic asphyxia, apparently being inhibited by central mechanisms. Hyperpnea calls upon activity of these muscles at the end—and only at the end—of expiration (Campbell, 1958).

Voluntary Sphincters

Sphincter Ani Externus

The anal sphincter is in a state of tonic contraction (Floyd and Walls, 1953). The degree of this tone varies with posture and the subject's alertness, falling to a very low level during sleep. Presumably, the internal sphincter is the main agency for keeping the rectum closed during sleep. The contraction of the sphincter ani externus is not isolated but is accompanied by general contraction of the perineal muscles, especially the sphincter urethrae.

With increased intra-abdominal pressure produced by straining, speaking, coughing, laughing or weight-lifting, increased sphincteric activity is related in amount to the degree of pressure. However, actual efforts to defaecate are usually (but not always) accompanied by relaxation of the sphincter ani.

Sphincter Urethrae

When the bladder is empty, its striated-muscle sphincter is relatively inactive. As the bladder fills slowly, activity increases and there is a continuous low level of activity as long as the bladder contains fluid. Activity disappears as micturition begins, and remains absent if the bladder is empty. Sudden voluntary stopping of micturition before the bladder is empty is accompanied by a marked outburst of potentials, which subsides rapidly to the resting level.

In women, the pelvic floor, or pelvic diaphragm, is mostly muscular and is very important in parturition. The pubococcygeal part of levator ani shows constant activity even in the occasional women who can relax the sphincter urethrae (Petersén et al., 1955, 1962). Diminution or complete cessation of activity in the sphincter urethrae at micturition (or attempted micturition) agrees with our findings in men. Voluntary efforts to contract the one muscle automatically recruit the contraction of the others.

REFERENCES

Bearn, J. G. (1961). The significance of the activity of the abdominal muscles in weight lifting. *Acta anat.*, *45:* 83–89.

Boyd, W. H. and Basmajian, J. V. (1963). Electromyography of the diaphragm in rabbits. *Am. J. Physiol.*, *204:* 943–948.

Campbell, E. J. M. (1958). *The Respiratory Muscles and the Mechanics of Breathing*, Lloyd-Luke (Medical Books) Ltd., London.

Fick, R. (1911). *Handbuch der Anatomie und Mechanik der Gelenke*, vol. 3. Gustav Fischer, Jena, Germany.

Flint, M. M. (1965). An electromyographic comparison of the function of the iliacus and the rectus abdominis muscles. A preliminary report. *J. Am. Phys. Therap. Assoc.*, *45:* 248–253.

Floyd, W. F. and Walls, E. W. (1953). Electromyography of the sphincter ani externus in man. *J. Physiol.*, *122:* 599–609.

Hoover, F. (1922). The functions and integration of the intercostal muscles. *Arch. Int. Med.*, *30:* 1–33.

Jones, D. S., Beargie, R. J. and Pauly, J. E. (1953). An electromyographic study of some muscles of costal respiration in man. *Anat. Rec.*, *117:* 17–24.

Morris, J. M., Lucas, D. B. and Bresler, B. (1961). The role of the trunk in stability of the spine. Publication no. 42. Biomechanics Laboratory, University of California, Berkeley.

Murphy, A. J., Koepke, G. H., Smith, E. M. and Dickinson, D. C. (1959). Sequence of action of the diaphragm and intercostal muscles during respiration. II. Expiration. *Arch. Phys. Med.*, *40:* 337–342.

Petersén, I., Franksson, C. and Danielsson, C.-O. (1955). Electromyographic study of the muscles of the pelvic floor and urethra in normal females. *Acta Obst. et Gynec. Scandinav.*, *34:* 273–285.

Petersén, I., Stener, I., Selldén, U. and Kollberg, S. (1962). Investigation of urethral sphincter in women with simultaneous electromyography and micturition urethro-cystography. *Acta Neurol. Scandinav.*, *suppl. 3*, *38:* 145–151.

Raper, A. J., Thompson, W. T., Jr., Shapiro, W. and Patterson, J. S., Jr. (1966). Scalene and sternomastoid muscle function. *J. Appl. Physiol.*, *21:* 497–502.

Sheffield, F. J. (1962). Electromyographic study of the abdominal muscles in walking and other movements. *Am. J. Phys. Med.*, *41:* 142–147.

Steindler, A. (1955). *Kinesiology of the Human Body under Normal and Pathological Conditions*, Charles C Thomas, Springfield, Ill.

Strasser, H. (1913). *Lehrbuch der Muskel und Gelenkmeckanik*, J. Springer, Berlin.

Taylor, A. (1960). The contribution of the intercostal muscles to the effort of respiration in man. *J. Physiol. 151:* 390–402.

ELEVEN

Pectoral Girdle, Arm and Forearm

The joints of the pectoral or shoulder girdle are the sterno-clavicular, coracoclavicular and acromioclavicular. Many movements which appear to occur in the glenohumeral joint really occur in these joints. Without their contribution, movement of the upper limb is seriously restricted.

The clavicle is the only bone of the upper limb that is joined firmly to the axial skeleton. Although the strut-like qualities of the clavicle are well known and although the transmission of forces from arm to scapula to clavicle to sternum is vital (fig. 11.1), the mooring effect of muscles attaching the scapula and shoulder area to the trunk cannot be ignored (fig. 11.2).

The scapula lies buried among the muscles that cover the upper part of the back of the thorax where it is shifted around and steadied by these muscles. Because the sternoclavicular joint lies in front of the thorax, the extremely varied movements of the upper limb are largely carried out in front of the body. In conformity with this the scapula lies, not in a coronal plane, but in a plane about midway between the coronal and sagittal. It lies against the curved, barrel-shaped thoracic cage and slides about on a bed of areolar tissue and muscle. Obviously the shape of the thorax and the clavicular attachments constrain the movements of the scapula.

The upper limb girdle has maximized mobility while sacri-

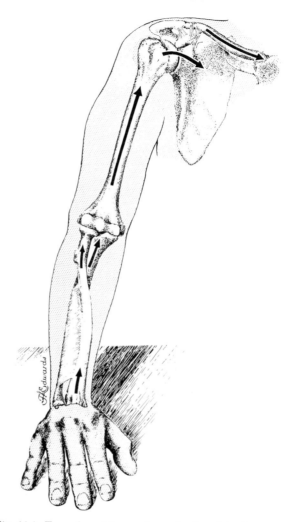

Fig. 11.1. Transfer of forces from the hand to the sternum.

ficing a large measure of stability. Thus the ligaments of the clavicle allow movements in some directions while preventing or limiting movements in others. The various ligaments have, in general, a unity of direction. However, only one function is shared by all—transmission of forces from the arm to the

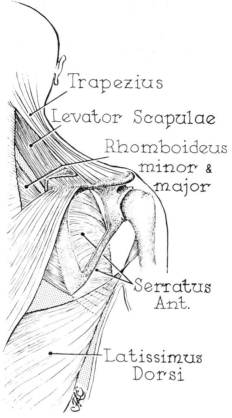

Fig. 11.2. The mooring muscles of the scapula are dynamic ligaments.

sternum. In addition, the ligaments have other individual functions to perform.

DEFINITIONS. The scapula gives attachment to many muscles. It can be braced back in a highly "military" position, when its vertebral border lies parallel to and approaches the vertebral spines; then the bone is said to be *retracted*. Or, it can be slid forward round the curved chest wall to an excessively "round-shouldered" position when its vertebral border lies far distant from the vertebral spines; then the bone is said to be *protracted*. As protraction proceeds, the vertebral border assumes a less and less vertical position since the inferior angle of the bone travels considerably faster than any other part. In other words, the scapula. is *rotated* so that the socket of the shoulder joint (glenoid cavity) looks more upwards. This combination of rotation with protraction is a desirable feature because it is the position demanded by the hands when they carry out their many duties in front of the body and at, or or near, eye level.

Besides these movements of retraction, protraction and rotation, the scapula can be *elevated* (shrugging the shoulders) or *depressed* (drooping shoulders). Elevation is commonly, though by no means invariably, accompanied by rotation of the scapula upwards, and is a relatively extensive movement. Depression is exceedingly limited, since, very early in the movement, the clavicle comes in contact with the first rib and cannot permit the scapula to sink farther.

Sternoclavicular Joint

In every one of the above-mentioned scapular movements the sternoclavicular joint is vitally concerned. It lies at the apex of an imaginary cone (fig. 11.3). The circumference of the base of this cone is described by the lateral end of the clavical, which can sweep in a circle. While the lateral end of the bone sweeps at will in the arcs of many circles, the medial end has

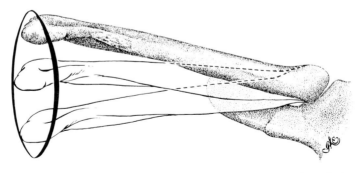

Fig. 11.3. The lateral end of the clavicle describes a sweeping circle which is the base of a cone, the apex of which is at the sternoclavicular joint.

merely to glide in its socket. The clavicle thus functions to hold the shoulder joint at its proper distance from the mid-line; it is a strut. A blow on the side of the shoulder or a fall on the outstretched arm imparts its force to the clavicle which transmits it to the axial skeleton at the sternoclavicular joint.

The joint surface on the sternum is concave from above downwards but slightly convex from front to back. The joint surface on the medial end of the clavicle is not reciprocally shaped; it is rather flat and only slightly convex. The contact of the otherwise ill-fitting surfaces is improved by the exist-ence of a disc, which however is much more occupied with the duties of absorbing the forces transmitted to the joint along the clavicle from the shoulder region and preventing the clavicle from being driven out of its socket on the sum-mit of the sternum. The disc can discharge these duties be-cause it is firmly attached—above, to the clavicle; below, to the first costal cartilage. The rarity of dislocation of the joint testifies to the efficiency of the disc in discharging its duties— even when a hole is worn in its middle with advanced age. The disc also aids the effective lubrication of the joint.

Excessive protraction and elevation of the clavicle are pre-vented by the existence of two structures, one a ligament, the other a muscle. Immediately lateral to the sternoclavicular joint, the clavicle is bound to the first costal cartilage by the rhomboidal costoclavicular ligament which, being near the centre of movement and at first somewhat lax, allows the lateral end of the clavicle considerable excursion in both pro-traction and elevation before it finally becomes so taut as to bring further movement to a halt. Lateral to the ligament is subclavius muscle which acts as a dynamic ligament (fig. 11.4).

Coracoclavicular and Acromioclavicular Joints

The lateral part of the clavicle crosses immediately above the right-angled bend in the coracoid process. At that site— located in the living at the hollow immediately below the lateral third of the clavicle—the strong coracoclavicular liga-

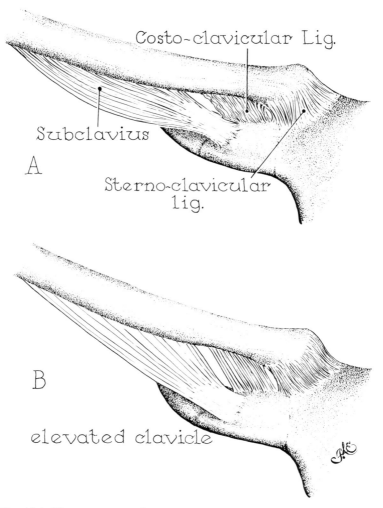

Fig. 11.4. The restraining ligaments of the medial end of the clavicle are reinforced by a "dynamic ligament," the subclavius muscle.

ment unites the under surface of the clavicle to the bend in the coracoid process (fig. 11.5). The result is a fibrous joint of considerable strength and, because the ligament has length, it allows some independent movement between the two bones;

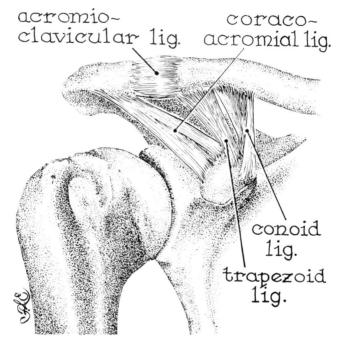

acromio-
clavicular lig.   coraco-
                 acromial lig.

conoid
lig.

trapezoid
lig.

Fig. 11.5. Ligaments of the coracoid process. The conoid and trapezoid
are two parts of the coracoclavicular.

but the union ensures that in all movements of any considerable extent the clavicle and scapula shall travel together.
Further, owing to the special oblique direction of its fibres,
the ligament transmits forces applied to the scapula at the
shoulder region, to and along the strong and prismatic medial
two-thirds of the clavicle.

At the lateral end of the clavicle is the small acromioclavicular joint. It is here that the scapula moves upon the clavicle
and that the true centre of rotation of the scapula lies. It
takes little or no part in the transmission of force to the clavicle
until it comes into or near the close-packed position. This
occurs at a later stage in the unloaded arm but quite early
(after some 20° of forward rotation) in the scapula when the

hand is carrying a load of 5 lbs. From the position of close-pack onwards the scapulo-clavicular complex moves as a whole in the sternoclavicular joint, and the coraco-clavicular ligaments are fully stretched. The arm then hangs from a "hook", the shank of which is formed by the clavicle and the crook of which is composed of the acromial process, the spine of the scapula and the base of the coracoid process (which forms part of the glenoid fossa). This joint also has an intra-articular disc. It is incomplete and is placed where the maximum pressure stress occurs between the bones during movement. Like such discs elsewhere it aids in lubrication.

Muscles and Movements of the Shoulder Girdle

In static loading, the upper fibres of trapezius, contrary to the universal teaching, "play no active part in the support of the shoulder girdle in the relaxed upright posture" (Bearn, 1961). Some persons initially show a low level of activity in this part of the trapezius, but upon their being instructed to relax, the activity stops entirely.

A low level of activity in trapezius (upper), levator scapulae and serratus anterior (upper) is sufficient to suspend the girdle, but when a weight is either supported on the shoulder or carried in the hand these muscles contract vigorously. Apparently, even with considerable loading, relaxation of trapezius is possible in many persons. One can only surmise that the clavicle is then suspended by the first rib and ligaments at the sternoclavicular joint—all these being passive structures.

SIMPLE DEPRESSION of the shoulder girdle may be brought about by the weight of the limb. But as an active movement, e.g., pressing downward or resting on parallel bars, it calls into action the pectoralis minor, which acts on the girdle, and the pectoralis major and latissimus dorsi, which act on the humerus (fig. 11.6). When one falls on one's outstretched hand, the timely contraction of these muscles saves the clavicle from fracture (fig. 11.1).

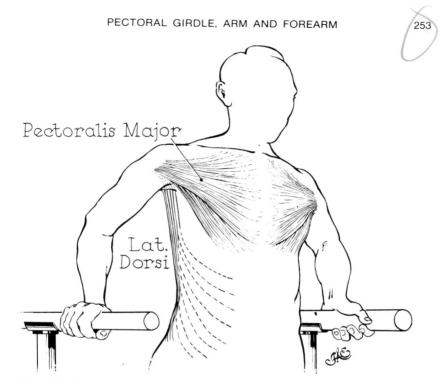

Pectoralis Major

Lat.
Dorsi

Fig. 11.6. Though inserted on the humerus, two large muscles pull down on the shoulder girdle.

ELEVATION WITH UPWARD ROTATION OF GLENOID CAVITY. In this movement the acromion rises, the superior angle of the scapula descends, and the inferior angle swings laterally. This movement is almost always part of a larger movement involving either abduction or flexion of the shoulder joint, as when the hand reaches for some object above the head, *i.e.*, the entire limb is elevated.

Just as scapular rotation is a distinct and important function, well-known for a century, so the muscles which produce the movement are a distinct functional group. The upper part of trapezius, the levator scapulae and the upper digits of serratus anterior constitute a unit whose main activities are in concert: they passively support the scapula (slight continuous activity), elevate it (increasing activity) and act as the upper component of a force couple that rotates the scapula (figs. 11.7, 11.8).

The lower part of trapezius and lower half or more of the serratus anterior constitute the lower component of the scapular rotatory force couple; they act with increasing vigour throughout elevation of the arm. The lower part of trapezius is the more active component of the lower force couple during abduction, but in flexion it is less active than serratus anterior,

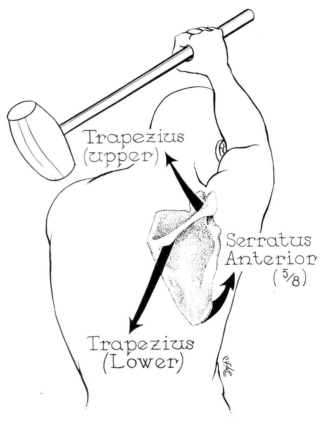

Fig. 11.7. The force-couple that rotates the scapula upward.

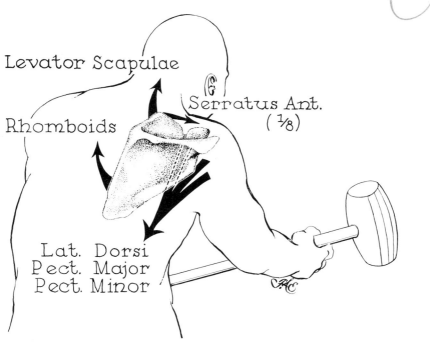

Levator Scapulae

Serratus Ant.
(⅛)

Rhomboids

Lat. Dorsi
Pect. Major
Pect. Minor

Fig. 11.8. The force-couple that rotates the scapula downward.

apparently because the scapula must be pulled forward during flexion.

The middle fibres of trapezius are most active in abduction, especially as the arm reaches the horizontal plane (90°). In forward flexion, the activity of the middle fibres of trapezius decreases during the early range but builds up toward the end. In general, then, the middle trapezius serves to fix the scapula but must relax to allow the scapula to slide forward during the early part of flexion.

DEPRESSION WITH DOWNWARD ROTATION OF GLENOID CAVITY, *i.e.*, recovering from the last movement or overstepping the recovery, as in chopping wood (fig. 11.8): the pectoralis minor, rhomboids, levator scapulae and trapezius (especially the middle portion) are called into play, and the pectoralis major and latissimus dorsi, which act indirectly through the humerus, give them powerful assistance.

Protraction of the scapula or forward movement, *e.g.*, pushing: the serratus anterior, pectoralis minor and levator scapulae act together with the pectoralis major.

Retraction of the scapula or backward movement, *i.e.*, recovering from the last movement or overstepping the recovery (*e.g.*, pulling): the trapezius (middle portion) and the rhomboids act with the latissimus dorsi. The last-named exerts an important associated backward and downward pull on the humerus to which it runs.

Although the rhomboids and the serratus are antagonistic in that they pull the scapula in opposite directions, they work together in holding the medial border of the scapula applied to the thoracic wall. The levator scapulae arises from transverse processes and therefore draws the scapula upward and forward; the rhomboids arise from spinous processes and therefore draw it upward and backward.

SHOULDER JOINT

The shoulder joint enjoys a remarkable degree of freedom of movement. It is a loose union between two mobile bones and its extreme mobility has been achieved only at the expense of stability and security, dislocation of the joint being a common accident.

Movements of the shoulder joint should not be confused with movements of the shoulder region. The two very commonly occur together but in any analysis of muscular activities it is helpful to segregate them, since movements of the shoulder region primarily involve the clavicle and scapula, whereas movements of the shoulder joint occur solely between the scapula and the humerus.

ARTICULAR SURFACES. The glenoid cavity of the scapula faces as much forwards as it does lateralward (fig. 11.9). It is shallowly concave and of much smaller area than the head of the humerus. The addition of a rim of fibro-cartilage to its peri-

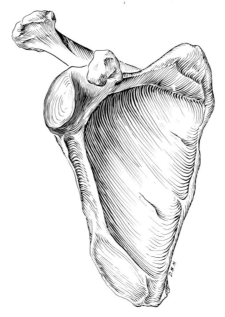

Fig. 11.9. Correct orientation of the scapula (here viewed directly from in front at eye level).

phery—the labrum—slightly deepens that socket but adds little to the security of the joint. The area of actual contact between the two bones is never very great and a considerable amount of the head of the humerus is at all times in contact with a lax part of the capsule (figs. 11.10, 11.11).

CAPSULE AND LIGAMENTS. No other important joint has such a loose capsule and is so ill-equipped with restraining ligaments. The only one worthy of a name is the coracohumeral ligament, and it extends from the coracoid process to the greater tuberosity of the humerus. Only its anterior edge is free, the remainder blending with, and thickening, the upper part of the fibrous capsule. The ligament becomes taut on lateral rotation. This ligament, along with the superior part of the capsule, is also taut when the arm hangs vertically. In company with supraspinatus muscle, it prevents downward

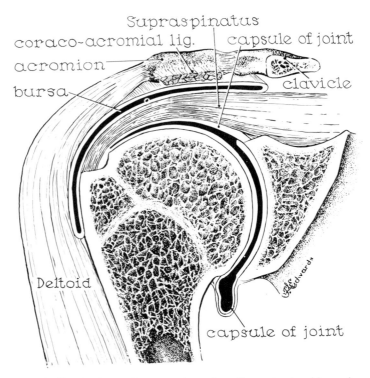

Supraspinatus

coraco-acromial lig.   capsule of joint

acromion

bursa

clavicle

Deltoid

capsule of joint

Fig. 11.10. Semi-schematic coronal section through shoulder when arm is hanging.

dislocation of the humeral head (see below). The anterior part of the capsule contains three thickenings—the gleno-humeral ligaments—which are of doubtful significance.

Whatever security the joint possesses during most of its excursion derives, not from ligaments, but from the muscles that surround and move it. Of these, four, as they pass to their insertions on the two tuberosities immediately adjacent to the head of humerus, blend with the capsule and so re-inforce it. By this device the capsule is reinforced in front, above and behind; its weakest site remains below. (The tendon of the long head of the biceps lies in the groove between the two tuberosities, having traversed the upper part of the in-

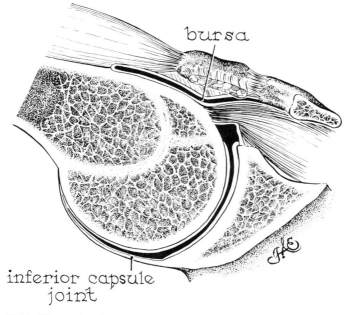

Fig. 11.11. When the humerus is raised, the lower part of the capsule becomes taut.

terior of the joint; perhaps it lends additional security by aiding in holding the head of the humerus in its socket.)

Coraco-Acromial Arch

The coracoid process in front and the acromion above and behind are united to one another by the thin, flat and triangular coraco-acromial ligament (fig. 11.5). Coracoid, ligament and acromion together may be called the secondary socket, and they form a continuous protective arch above the shoulder joint. Immediately under the coraco-acromial arch lies the tendon of supraspinatus muscle blended with the capsule of the shoulder joint. To reduce friction between the tendon and the arch a large bursa—the subacromial bursa—is interposed (figs. 11.10, 11.11).

Movements and Muscles of the Glenohumeral Joint

The joint may be flexed, extended, abducted, adducted and rotated (medially or laterally). Any movements that elevate the arm above the level of the shoulder involve extensive scapular and clavicular movements as well. Indeed, it is probable that most movements of the humerus call for some concomitant movement of the glenoid cavity even before the horizontal plane is reached.

The chief muscles that act upon the shoulder (glenohumeral) joint are the deltoid, the pectorales, the latissimus dorsi, teres major and the four rotator cuff muscles—subscapularis, supraspinatus, infraspinatus and teres minor.

ABDUCTION. The obvious activity in the deltoid increases progressively and become greatest between 90° and 180° of elevation (fig. 11.12); the activity of supraspinatus increases progressively, too—it is not simply an initiator of abduction as was formerly taught. Complete experimental paralysis of supraspinatus in man simply reduces the force of abduction and power of endurance. In abduction, supraspinatus plays only a quantitative and not a specialized rôle. No part of pectoralis major is active during abduction. The rôle of biceps brachii in abduction seems to be confined to a contribution in maintaining this position while the arm is laterally rotated and the forearm supine. When the arm is medially rotated and the forearm prone, biceps does not contribute to abduction.

FLEXION. The clavicular head of pectoralis major along with the anterior fibres of deltoid are the chief flexors; the former reaches its maximum activity at 115° of flexion. Both heads of biceps brachii are active in flexion of the shoulder joint, the long head being the more active.

DEPRESSORS OF HUMERUS. Subscapularis, infraspinatus and teres minor form a functional group which acts as the second or inferior group of the force couple during abduction of the humerus. They act continuously during both abduction and

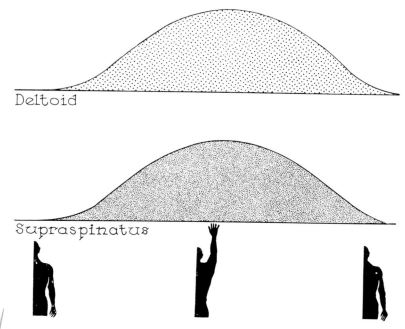

Fig. 11.12. Schematic representation of EMG activity during abduction of the shoulder joint.

flexion. In abduction, activity in infraspinatus and teres minor rises linearly, while activity in subscapularis reaches a peak or plateau beyond the 90° angle and then falls off.

ADDUCTION. Pectoralis major and latissimus dorsi produce adduction. The posterior fibres of deltoid are also very active, perhaps to resist the medial rotation that the main adductors would produce if unresisted.

TERES MAJOR. Teres major never exhibits activity during motion, coming into action only when it is necessary to maintain a static position (Inman et al., 1944). In static positions, it reaches its maximum activity at about 90°. Even during the vigorous activity of shot-putting, the teres major remains relatively quiet (Hermann, 1962).

LATISSIMUS DORSI. Medial rotation of the humerus is performed by this muscle when it may be more important than pectoralis major, the latter muscle becoming active when rotation is resisted. As noted before, it also depresses and retracts the scapula.

DELTOID. The three parts of deltoid are active in all movements of the arm. In flexion and medial rotation, the anterior part is more active than the posterior; in extension and lateral rotation, the posterior is the more active; and in abduction the middle part is the most active. While one part of deltoid is acting as the prime mover, the other parts may be stabilizing the joint in the glenoid cavity.

The posterior part has its principal action in extension, but the action is inconstant and slight in abduction and elevation of the arm. Its participation in lateral rotation is minimal, being practically absent. It also becomes active during heavy downward pulls on the humerus as part of a locking mechanism at the shoulder joint (see below).

Prevention of Downward Dislocation of the Humerus

Except for its posterior fibres, deltoid (the muscle one would expect to be especially active in preventing downward dislocation of the humerus) is inactive even with heavy pulls (Basmajian and Bazant, 1959). Other muscles running vertically from the scapula to the humerus, particularly the biceps and the long head of triceps, are conspicuously inactive as well. Therefore, downward dislocation is prevented by the superior part of the capsule along with the supraspinatus (and to a lesser extent the posterior fibres of the deltoid) although these structures run in a horizontal and not in a vertical direction. The underlying mechanism, which is described fully in Chapter 8 (p. 192), cannot operate when there is abduction of the humerus. As a result, the head can be easily subluxated when it is in the abducted position in the cadaver and in anesthetized normal man.

In conscious persons, the muscles that prevent dislocation

of the joint in its unstable position are the "rotator cuff" muscles—supraspinatus, infraspinatus, teres minor and sub-scapularis (and perhaps teres major and other muscles spanning the joint).

Swinging of the Arm during Gait

In normal persons, the posterior and middle parts of deltoid begin to show activity slightly before the arm starts its backward swing, and this continues throughout the backward swing. The upper part of latissimus dorsi and the teres major act from the onset of the backward swing until the arm reaches the line of the body.

During forward swing of the arm, activity is confined to some of the medial rotators; the main flexors are strikingly silent. Apart from brief silent periods in the extreme positions of swing, trapezius is active in both phases to maintain elevation of the shoulder. Similar activity occurs in supraspinatus; this obviously is related to the prevention of downward dislocation, already discussed.

ELBOW JOINT

Although the elbow joint proper is the hinge joint between the lower end of the humerus and the upper ends of the ulna and radius, the superior radio-ulnar joint is closely associated with it. They share one capsule and their joint spaces are continuous. Indeed, we would not discuss one without the other.

The jaws of the deep trochlear notch on the face of the spanner-like upper end of the ulna grasp the trochlea of the lower end of the humerus. This trochlea resembles an hour-glass laid on its side, the medial end of the hour-glass having a greater circumference than the lateral.

CARRYING ANGLE. As the ulna swings round the trochlea from flexion to extension the difference between the two ends of the hour-glass makes itself felt and is responsible for the ulna being forced gradually lateralwards and so out of line with the humerus. This difference in alignment between humerus and ulna amounts, when the elbow is fully extended, to about 15°. It is compensated for when the lower end of the radius crosses over to the medial side of the ulna, the angularity of the extended and supinated limb disappearing on pronation.

The radius and the ulna lie side by side, but the radius reaches only as high as the coronoid process of the ulna which forms the lower part of the trochlear notch. The circumference of the disc-like head of the radius turns against the hollow on the lateral side of the coronoid process, the radial notch of the ulna; this is less than one-quarter of the circumference of the radial head that can articulate with it at any one time. The remainder of the circumference is accomodated by the anular ligament, which is of smaller circumference below than above; thus it tends to prevent the radius from being pulled down out of its socket.

The upper surface of the radial head is circular in outline and slightly concave and, when accompanying the ulna in movements of flexion and extension, moves on the capitulum situated immediately lateral to the trochlea.

COLLATERAL LIGAMENTS AND CAPSULE. The medial ligament spreads from medial epicondyle to the medial edge of the trochlear notch of the ulna; its anterior part is thickened to form a cord which plays the biggest part in the prevention of abduction at the elbow. The lateral ligament runs from lateral epicondyle to the outer surface of the anular ligament and so does not impede supination and pronation. Since the anular ligament grasps the head of the radius firmly in the adult, adduction is effectively prohibited by the lateral ligament.

Elbow Flexors

The biceps brachii, the brachialis and the brachioradialis are primarily concerned with flexion. A variety of theories have obscured the rôle played by each during flexion and other movements of the elbow. Actually, in the movements produced by the flexors there is a fine interplay among them and a wide range of response from person to person. Thus there is no unanimity of action. For example, the brachialis is generally markedly active during quick flexion of the supine forearm, but occasionally it is completely inactive.

There is an irregular selection in the sequence of appearance and disappearance of activity in these muscles. Any one may function first or last in an unpredictable fashion, i.e., there is no set pattern. In the same way, the activity ceases in the muscles in an unpredictable order. Moreover, the muscles that show the greatest activity in individual subjects only occasionally begin first and end last.

The long head of the biceps generally shows more activity than the short head during slow flexion of the forearm, during supination of the forearm against resistance and during flexion of the shoulder joint (although there is little difference between the activity of the two heads during isometric contraction and during extension of the elbow).

The biceps is generally active during flexion of the supine forearm under all conditions and during flexion of the semiprone forearm when a load of approximately a kilogram is lifted (fig. 11.13). However with the forearm prone, in the majority of instances the biceps plays little if any rôle in flexion, in maintenance of elbow flexion and in antagonistic action during extension, even with a load. If the forearm is in supination, the biceps acts during flexion when there is only slight resistance, but in a position of complete pronation it does not act until the resistance is at least 4 lbs. (approximately 2 kilograms).

The biceps is usually described as a supinator of the forearm. However, no activity occurs in the muscle during supination of the extended forearm through the whole range of movement except when resistance to supination is given. Apparently because of the tendency of the biceps to flex the forearm, it is reflexly inhibited during ordinary supination;

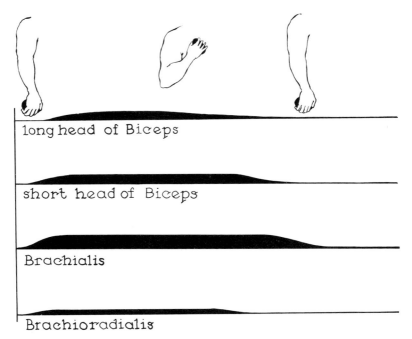

Fig. 11.13. Schematic representation of EMG activity during slow flexion of the elbow while holding a load in the hand.

thus position of the forearm is maintained while the supinator does the supinating. On the other hand, when supination is resisted, the biceps comes into strong action; usually the previously extended forearm is partly flexed as well during supination against resistance.

The brachialis has been generally and erroneously considered to be a muscle of speed rather than one of power because of its short leverage. Yet it is a flexor of the supine, semiprone and prone forearm in both slow and quick flexion, and either with or without an added weight, apparently because the line of its pull does not change with pronation or supination.

Maintenance of specific flexed postures of the elbow, *i.e.*, isometric contraction, and the movement of slow extension (when the flexors must act as anti-gravity muscles) both generally bring the brachialis into activity in all positions of the forearm. This is not the case with the other two flexor muscles. Thus, one might call the brachialis the "workhorse" among the flexor muscles of the elbow.

A short burst of activity is generally seen in all the muscles during quick extension. This activity can hardly be considered antagonistic in the usual sense. Rather, it may provide a protective function for the joint.

In the past, the brachioradialis has been described as a flexor, acting to its best advantage in the semiprone position of the forearm. Almost never does the brachioradialis play an appreciable rôle during maintenance of elbow flexion and during slow flexion and extension when the movement is carried out without a weight. When a weight is lifted during flexion, the brachioradialis is generally moderately active in the semiprone or prone position of the forearm and is slightly active in the supine position. There is no comparable increase in activity with the addition of weight during maintenance of flexion and during slow extension.

During both quick flexion and quick extension, the brachioradialis is quite active in all three positions of the forearm. It follows that the muscle is recruited for occasions when speedy movement is required and when weight is to be lifted, especially in the semiprone and the prone positions. In the latter position, the biceps usually does not come into prominent action. More important the activity of the brachioradialis in speedy movements is related to its function as a shunt muscle (p. 150).

The brachioradialis neither supinates nor pronates the extended forearm. When these movements are performed against resistance, brachioradialis acts only as an accessory muscle, or as a synergist.

While the biceps, brachialis and brachioradialis differ in their flexor activity in the three positions of the forearm (prone, semiprone and supine), all three act maximally when a weight is lifted during flexion of the semiprone forearm. The semiprone position of the forearm is the natural position of the forearm, the position of rest and the position of greatest advantage for most functions of the upper limb.

PRONATOR TERES AND ELBOW FLEXION. Pronator teres contributes to elbow flexion only when resistance is offered to the movement. It shows no activity during unresisted flexion whether the forearm is prone, semiprone or supine.

Triceps Brachii

The long head of triceps is surprisingly quiescent during active extension of the elbow regardless of the position of either the subject or his limb (Travill, 1962). The medial head, however, is always active and appears to be the prime extensor of the elbow; meanwhile, the lateral head shows some activity as well. Against resistance, the lateral and long heads are recruited. Therefore, we might compare the medial head of triceps to the brachialis which we noted above to be the workhorse of the elbow flexors; it is the workhorse of the extensors. The lateral and long heads are reserves for extension just as the two heads of biceps are reserves for flexion. The long head is less involved than the lateral one, probably owing to the lack of fixation of the scapular origin and the necessity of adducting the shoulder with the forearm either flexed or extended. Too strong a contribution from the long head would tend to give extension during adduction of the arm.

The *anconeus* should be regarded as an integral part of triceps with which it acts in extension.

THE FOREARM AND PRONATION-SUPINATION

The shafts of radius and ulna are united by an interosseous membrane (fig. 11.14) stretching between their adjacent sharp borders; the union is a fibrous joint and is sometimes called the intermediate radio-ulnar joint. The fibres of the membrane take a direction downwards and medialwards, a fact

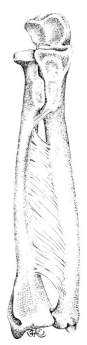

Fig. 11.14. The interosseous radio-ulnar ligament—the direction of its fibres is fortuitous.

which suggests that forces, received by the lower end of the radius from the hand, are transmitted on their passage up the forearm by the interosseous membrane to the ulna. This function of the membrane has been over-emphasized since the hand is usually in a position of pronation when forces are applied to it, and in pronation the interosseous membrane is rather slack. Moreover, there seems to be no good reason why the radius itself should be unable to transmit forces directly to the humerus. This has been shown to be the case (Travill, 1964). The more important use of the membrane would seem to be to increase the area available, both at the front and at the back, for the origins of the numerous muscles found in the forearm.

At the lower end of the two long bones of the forearm, the ulna is excluded from any participation in the wrist joint by a triangular plate of fibrocartilage lying immediately below its head, the articular disc, which is attached by its apex to the root of the styloid process. The base of the disc is attached to the radius along the lower margin of the ulnar notch. The apex of the disc is the centre of a circle, the arc of which is described by disc and radius in the movements of pronation and supination (fig. 11.15). This disc—which is a ligament—is an important agent for transfer of forces from the radius to the ulna. As elsewhere, the disc is important for the efficient lubrication called for by the flatness of the apposed part of the head of the ulna.

Muscles of Pronation and Supination

PRONATORS. Both pronator quadratus and pronator teres are active during pronation, the consistent prime pronating muscle being the pronator quadratus (fig. 11.16). This is true irrespective of the positions of the forearm in space or the angulation of the elbow joint. In general, the pronator teres

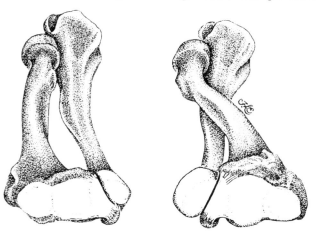

Fig. 11.15. The radius swings around the ulna on the fibrocartilaginous disc which joins their lower ends.

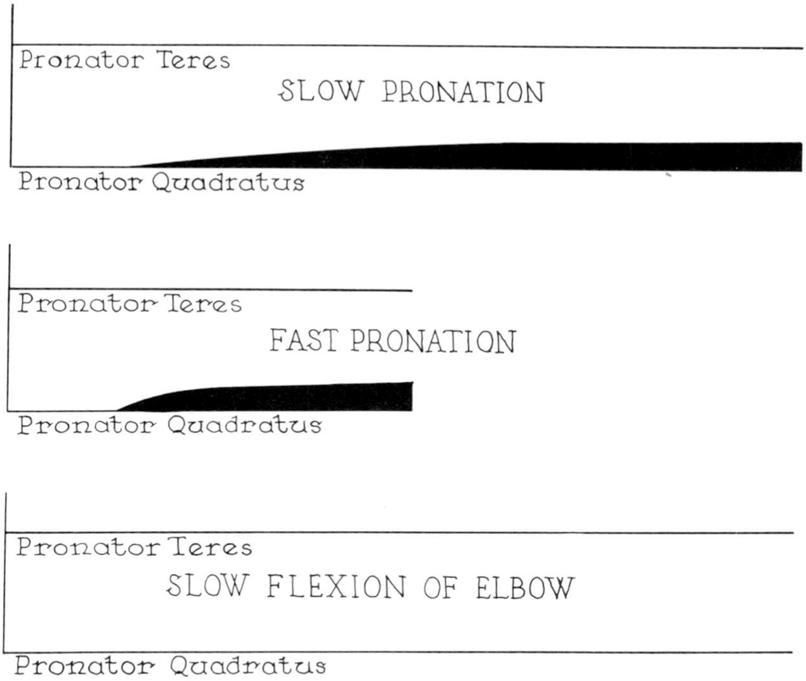

Pronator Teres

SLOW PRONATION

Pronator Quadratus

Pronator Teres

FAST PRONATION

Pronator Quadratus

Pronator Teres

SLOW FLEXION OF ELBOW

Pronator Quadratus

Fig. 11.16. Schematic representation of EMG activity in the pronator muscles during unresisted movements.

is called in as a reinforcing pronator whenever the action of pronation is rapid. Similar reinforcement occurs during pronation against resistance. Whether pronation is fast or slow, the activity in the pronator quadratus is markedly greater than that in the pronator teres. Regardless of whether the pronating action is carried out swiftly or slowly, the angle of the elbow joint has no bearing on the amount of activity of the pronator teres.

During slow supination there is no activity whatsoever in either of the pronators—though some have suggested that the deeper layer of the pronator quadratus acts as a supinator. The flexor carpi radialis, brachioradialis and extensor carpi ulnaris have no pronating function.

SUPINATORS. Brachioradialis (known for years as "supinator longus") is not a true supinator. Slow unresisted supination, whatever the position of the forearm, is brought about by the independent action of the supinator alone. Similarly, fast supination in the extended position requires only the supinator, but fast unresisted supination with the elbow flexed is assisted by the action of the biceps. All movements of forceful supination against resistance require the cooperation of the biceps during resisted supination, especially when the elbow is flexed.

Both the supinator muscles are completely relaxed during pronation (slow, fast or resisted). This is similar to our findings for pronation, where complete relaxation of the pronator quadratus and the pronator teres during supination is the rule.

The "hold" or static position of supination depends on activity in supinator for the maintenance of the supine posture. Against added resistance, however, the biceps always becomes active. The movement of supination is initiated, and mostly maintained, by the supinator; it is assisted by the biceps only as needed to overcome added resistance.

REFERENCES

Basmajian, J. V. and Bazant, F. J. (1959). Factors preventing downward dislocation of the adducted shoulder joint: an electromyographic and morphological study. *J. Bone and Joint Surg.*, *41-A:* 1182–1186.

Bearn, J. G. (1961). An electromyographic study of the trapezius, deltoid, pectoralis major, biceps and triceps muscles, during static loading of the upper limb. *Anat. Rec.*, *140:* 103–108.

Hermann, G. W. (1962). An electromyographic study of selected muscles involved in the shot put. *Res. Quart.*, *33:* 1–9.

Inman, V. T., Saunders, J. B. deC. M. and Abbott, L. C. (1944). Observations on the function of the shoulder joint. *J. Bone and Joint Surg.*, *26:* 1–30.

Travill, A. A. (1962). Electromyographic study of the extensor apparatus of the forearm. *Anat. Rec.*, *144:* 373–376.

Travill, A. A. (1964). Transmission of pressures across the elbow joint. *Anat. Rec.*, *150:* 243–247.

TWELVE

Wrist and Hand

Axial Line and Force Transmission

From all points of view, it soon became apparent that the middle finger, the third metacarpal and the capitate are the axial bones of the hand. To this axis forces are gathered, and around it many fine movements of the hand take place (fig. 12.1). The large capitate supports the base of the third metacarpal and, in part, those of the second and fourth. The second metacarpal (the most fixed) is supported by three carpals—capitate, trapezoid and trapezium. The fourth metacarpal is supported mainly, the fifth entirely, by the hamate which transmits its forces—not to the triquetrum—but to the lunate. Thus the force of a blow struck by any of the knuckles is transmitted to the radius. It is apparent, too, that the second and third metacarpals are in the most direct line of force transmission and are, therefore, the most efficient of the four for the delivery of a blow. Furthermore, the ligaments binding the adjacent carpal bones to the capitate take a direction designed to gather forces to this large, central and axial bone (fig. 12.2).

Wrist and Midcarpal Joints

The midcarpal joint acts as a hinge joint and therefore is in itself capable merely of flexion and extension. It moves in

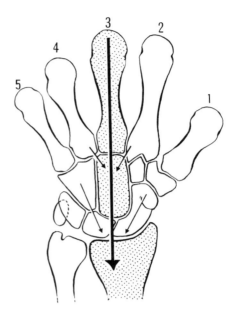

Fig. 12.1. Forces are gathered to the axis of the hand.

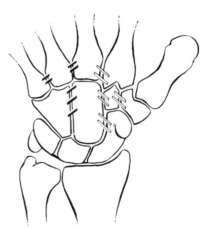

Fig. 12.2. Ligaments in the carpal region are so placed as to concentrate forces on the capitate.

conjunction with flexion and extension of the wrist joint to increase the range of these movements for the hand as a whole. In full dorsiflexion, the wrist joint is close-packed When wrist abduction and adduction occur, the midcarpal joint by its sinuosity locks the distal row to the proximal row and so ensures that the hand shall move as a whole (fig. 12.3); however, the two rows move sinuously upon each other be-

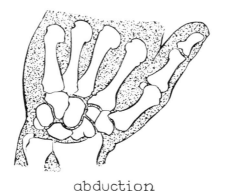

abduction

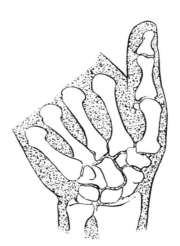

adduction

Fig. 12.3. The midcarpal joint during abduction and adduction.

cause of a sideways rotation of the capitate, keeping the other bones quite close together.

Carpometacarpal Joints

Of the joints at the bases of metacarpals, only that at the base of the thumb or first metacarpal possesses any considerable range of movement. At that joint, the metacarpal of the thumb articulates with the trapezium by means of the best example of a saddle joint to be found in the body. As has been remarked before, a saddle joint permits angular movements in any plane and a restricted amount of axial rotation (fig. 12.4); but this rotation is not independent, being always consequent upon movement of one component upon the other in an arcuate path (Chapter 4).

THUMB MOVEMENTS. A cursory inspection will reveal that the thumb metacarpal is "set" differently from the others. As a result, while the fronts and the backs of the fingers look in the orthodox directions, *viz.*, forwards and backwards, the corresponding surfaces of the thumb look medialwards and lateralwards, *i.e.*, at right angles to the fingers. This fact has to be borne in mind in describing the movements of the

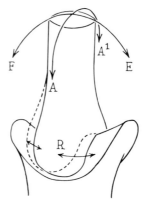

Fig. 12.4. Diagrammatic representation of the saddle joint at the base of the first metacarpal. A and A^1, abduction and adduction; E and F, extension and flexion; R, rotation.

thumb. For example, the movement that carries the thumb laterally away from fingers is extension. It should be noticed that the functional value of the thumb lies in its ability to be "opposed" to the fingers, and that the movement of opposition occurs at the saddle-shaped joint between the trapezium and first metacarpal.

METACARPAL MOVEMENTS. By passively manipulating the bases of the metacarpals it can be demonstrated that the mild degree of mobility enjoyed by the metacarpals of the little and ring fingers enables one to "cup" the hand and, perhaps, to improve the grip.

Metacarpophalangeal Joints

These are the joints between the heads of metacarpals and the bases of the first row of phalanges—the "knuckle joints". Of these joints, that of the thumb is the least mobile being similar to interphalangeal joints in function, though not in structure.

At the knuckle joint, a finger can be flexed until it is at right angles to the metacarpal or it can be extended somewhat beyond a straight line (*i.e.* slightly hyperextended). The articular cartilage on a metacarpal head needs to clothe the end and the palmar surface of the head, but it needs to extend for only a short distance on the dorsal surface. If the dried bone is examined, these are the dispositions found and, in addition, the articular surface is seen to be markedly convex from front to back but very much less so from side to side.

The base of a proximal phalanx has a small and slightly concave articular surface which is oval in outline with the long axis transverse.

PALMAR PLATES. Important tendons rub on the front of each joint and so the capsule becomes locally thickened to form a stiff plate of dense fibrous tissue known as a palmar plate or ligament (figs. 12.5, 12.6). It is attached to the anterior edge of the base of the phalanx, moving in consequence with the

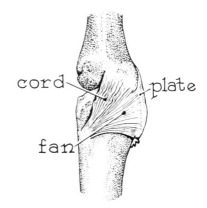

Fig. 12.5. A palmar plate and its ligaments.

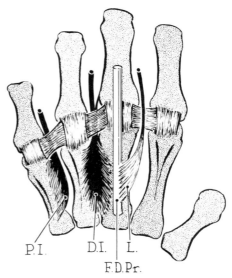

Fig. 12.6. The deep transverse ligament(s). The palmar and dorsal interossei (P.I. and D.I.) pass behind, the lumbricals (L.), in front; F.D.Pr. is a
long flexor tendon.

phalanx; it has only a loose attachment to the metacarpal.
The side of each plate is attached to its neighbour by a
square-shaped ligament; these ligaments are known as deep
transverse ligaments of the palm. The result is a fibrous band

stretching right across the palm and binding the metacarpal heads together (fig. 12.6). The palmar plate of the thumb has no such attachment to its neighbour but is free.

MOVEMENTS AND COLLATERAL LIGAMENTS OF FINGERS. When the fingers are extended they can be spread apart, but as they are flexed they are compelled finally to come together. The whole movement is an acquisitive one, the open hand to receive, the closed hand to clutch. Each side of each joint capsule is reinforced by a fan-shaped ligament rather particularly placed (fig. 12.5). The handle of the fan is attached to the side of the metacarpal head at a site which ensures that the ligament is completely taut on flexion but lax on extension; this is achieved by placing the attachment nearer the distal end than the palmar surface. From this site, the ligament fans out to the side of the base of the phalanx and to the palmar plate; the part to the phalanx is the stronger. These paired collateral ligaments prevent abduction and adduction of the flexed metacarpophalangeal joints. It is, in part, the function of these ligaments to bring together the fingers on making a fist. Muscles that control these movements are discussed on page 284.

Interphalangeal Joints

There are nine of these joints and each is a hinge of the purest variety. The head of each phalanx (except the terminal ones of course) is pulley-shaped, the base of the adjacent phalanx possessing a surface to match the two parts of the pulley. The device renders side to side movement impossible; hence the fingers can be flexed or extended, but no other movement occurs normally. The joints are reinforced with little collateral ligaments and equipped with palmar plates similar to those already met, but of course there can be no transverse ligaments uniting adjacent plates.

The thinnest part of the capsule of all metacarpophalangeal and all interphalangeal joints is at the back. Tendons on the back of the fingers, as they cross each joint in turn, flatten out and, blending with the capsule, afford it additional protection and security.

Extensors of Wrist

DISPOSITIONS. Only two layers of extensor muscles exist, a superficial and a deep. Even this statement needs qualifying for, halfway down the forearm, the superficial layer is split into a medial and a lateral group by the deep layer outcropping between them to become superficial also. When the fist is firmly clenched, the deep extensors can readily be recognized as a fleshy prominence running obliquely across the back of the radius near its lower end, and directed towards the thumb.

The superficial extensors, like the superficial flexors, are at first separated from one another only by intermuscular fibrous septa. They have a common origin from the lateral epicondyle of the humerus and consist of: extensor carpi radialis longus and extensor carpi radialis brevis which lower down become the lateral group; and extensor digitorum (communis), extensor digiti minimi and extensor carpi ulnaris which lower down become the medial group (fig. 12.7). The deep extensors come to the surface between the extensor carpi radialis brevis and the extensor digitorum.

EXTENSOR RETINACULUM. The extensor tendons occupy the lateral side as well as the back of the wrist and, lying in bony grooves, are held in place by a transverse band of fibrous tissue called the extensor retinaculum. From the deep surface of the extensor retinaculum a series of fibrous partitions pass to the margins of the bony grooves, and through six compartments thus produced run the 12 extensor tendons (fig. 12.8).

Functions of Extensors

Since the contributions that extensor digitorum itself makes to the extensor expansions can be traced no farther than the bases of the middle phalanges, the muscle can have no

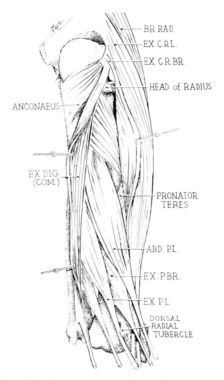

Fig. 12.7. Extensor muscles in the forearm.

power to extend the terminal phalanges. Indeed, its principal action is to extend the metacarpophalangeal joints and for them it is the sole extensor.

The extensores carpi ulnaris, radialis brevis and radialis longus extend the wrist and, acting with their companion flexors, produce side to side motion at the wrist (adduction and abduction).

Three deep out-cropping extensor muscles are almost exclusively devoted to what may properly be called "supination of the thumb". The movement is the contrary one to that performed when the thumb is "pronated" in order to oppose it to the other digits in such an everyday action as,

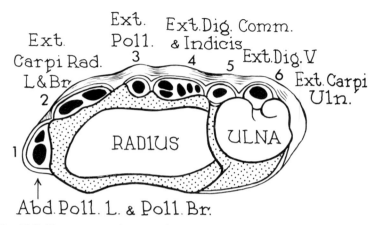

Fig. 12.8. Extensor tendons in their six compartments on the back of the wrist.

say, picking up a pencil. (A fourth and lowest muscle is present which joints the tendon of extensor digitorum of the index finger; it can, of course, produce only extension of the index.)

In a series from above downwards the out-cropping muscles to the thumb are abductor pollicis longus, extensor pollicis brevis and extensor pollicis longus (fig. 12.7). Their actions depend on the sites of insertion of their tendons and the direction of pull. Hold your wrist constantly straight with the palm facing the floor and draw the thumb laterally and backwards to point at the ceiling. Now the tendon of extensor pollicis longus will be seen running to its insertion on the dorsum of the base of the distal phalanx of the thumb, and jt can be traced back to the tubercle on the back of the lower end of the radius which it uses as a pulley to set the direction of its pull.

Next, stretch the thumb into the position of its widest span. This usually reveals the tendon of extensor pollicis brevis crossing the lateral aspect of the wrist (where it is held in a compartment of the extensor retinaculum) to its insertion on the base of the proximal phalanx.

Now, if the thumb is carried on through an arc until its tip stretches toward the floor, the tendon of abductor pollicis longus can be felt and seen as the most lateral tendon on the anterior aspect of the wrist. Its insertion is on the base of the first metacarpal. At the wrist, its tendon is in a compartment of the extensor retinaculum which is far enough forward for the muscle to abduct the thumb, to flex the wrist and to assist the extensors of the wrist and thumb in their stabilizing functions, one of the most significant being that of preventing the hand from being forced ulnarwards (as in holding a heavy jug by its handle).

Of the two radial extensors of the wrist the extensor carpi radialis brevis is much more active during pure extension than the longus whether the movement is slow or fast (Tournay and Paillard, 1953). Actually, except with fast extension, the longus is essentially inactive. However, the rôles of the two muscles are completely reversed during prehension or fist-making; now the longus is very active as a synergist. The two muscles are both quite active during abduction of the wrist, as one would guess from their positions.

During simple extension of the wrist there is a reciprocal innervation between extensors and flexors (Bäckdahl and Carlsöö, 1961). Extensores carpi radiales (longus et brevis) and extensor carpi ulnaris, as well as the extensor digitorum, work synchronously; none seems to be the prime mover. During forced extreme flexion of the wrist, there is a reactive co-contraction of the extensor carpi ulnaris, apparently to stabilize the wrist joint; this does not occur with the extensor digitorum and extensores carpi radiales.

Flexors of Wrist

There are six flexors in the forearm arranged in three layers, and the deeper the layer the more distal the insertions of its muscles. In general, the three flexors of this superficial layer act only on the wrist and carpal joints. As one would expect,

they are inserted—not on the mobile carpal bones—but on
the relatively fixed bases of the metacarpals. The one flexor
of the middle layer reaches the middle phalanges and acts on
all intermediate joints in passing. The two flexors of the deep
layer reach the terminal phalanges and similarly act on the
intermediate joints.

The flexor carpi radialis, palmaris longus and flexor carpi
ulnaris all flex the wrist, although the flexor palmaris longus
is not very powerful. The flexor carpi radialis is not an important abductor of the wrist; for that matter, the wrist can
be abducted very little from "neutral". But the flexor carpi
ulnaris is an important adductor, acting in concert with the
extensor carpi ulnaris.

All the muscles of the wrist are quite important for their
synergistic use in stabilizing the wrist so that the fingers and
fist work to best advantage.

During flexion of the wrist, the flexores carpi radialis, ulnaris and superficialis act synchronously,—none is the sole
prime mover. Flexor digitorum profundus plays no rôle. Two
possible muscles in the antagonist position (the radial extensors of the wrist and the extensors of the fingers) are passive,
even in extreme flexion of the wrist, but the extensor carpi
ulnaris shows marked activity as an antagonist.

In abduction and adduction, the appropriate flexors and
extensors act reciprocally as one might expect, the antagonist
muscles relaxing. Extensor digitorum contracts during abduction (radial abduction), but this contraction is not limited to
the radial part of the muscle, and the flexor digitorum superficialis may be active too. Apparently this type of activity
has a synergistic function. Similarly there is antagonist activity
in the flexors when the wrist is extended and the metacarpophalangeal joints hyperextended.

Fingers

When all the fingers are moving simultaneously the activity
of the "antagonist" muscles conforms to the principle of re-

ciprocal inhibition (Person and Roshtchina, 1958). When only the little finger or ring finger is moving while the others are extended, the extensor is active during both extension and flexion. When one finger is moved while the others are kept bent, the flexor is active during both movements. If a single finger moves, the "antagonist" must remain active to immobilize the other fingers. However, if the other fingers are held immobile by an observer, there is no activity in the antagonist muscle.

The lumbricals of the hand are important only in extension of the interphalangeal joints. It is now generally accepted that the importance of lumbrical-interosseus extension at the interphalangeal joints is in the prevention of hyperextension of the proximal phalanx by the extensor digitorum. This preventive action allows a more efficient pull on the dorsal expansion which extends the interphalangeal joints (fig. 12.9). These muscles are capable of bringing about the pronations necessary to bring them into their close-packed position, which is that of full extension.

Metacarpophalangeal flexion is performed by a lumbrical only when the interphalangeal joints are extended. A lumbrical has no effect on rotation or radial deviation of its finger during opposition with the thumb.

The extensor digitorum begins or increases its activity with the inception of interphalangeal (IP) joint extension regardless of the position of the metacarpophalangeal (MP) joints, and even with moderate effort. During extension or hyperextension of the MP joint, extensor digitorum alone is active.

Flexor digitorum superficialis is active during flexion of the middle phalanx (proximal IP joint), and it is active in flexion of the MP joint providing the next distal joint is stabilized. Surprisingly, the superficialis is active during rapid, forceful IP extension regardless of the position of the MP joint.

The interossei act as MP flexors only when their other action of IP extension does not conflict (Long, 1968). Therefore they act best and strongest when combined MP-flexion—IP-

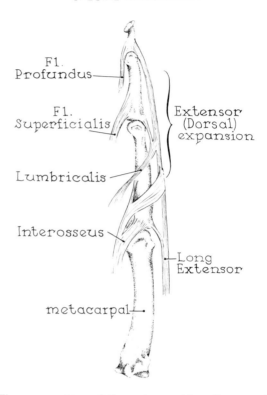

Fig. 12.9. The composition of the extensor (dorsal) expansion of a finger.

extension is performed. During all IP extension, the intrinsic muscles of the hand contract regardless of MP posture.

The long tendons of the fingers provide the gross motion of opening and closing of the fist at all the joints simultaneously. However, the intrinsic muscles perform their major function during any departure from this simple total opening or closing movement. Thus, they are the primary IP extensors while the MP joints are flexing.

Neither the interossei nor the lumbricals of one finger act during closing of the full hand, suggesting that in this total movement they are not synergists.

The activity of the long extensors and flexors occurs in

special sequences. Extensor digitorum acts during MP extension—in both the movement and the "hold" position. But it
is also active in many flexion movements of that joint, apparently acting as a brake. The flexor profundus is the most
consistently active flexor of the finger. Joined by the flexor
superficialis, the profundus may act as a secondary flexor
of the wrist joint also. The superficialis has its maximal action when the hand is being closed or held closed without
flexion of the distal IP joint.

Thenar and Hypothenar Muscles

Each of the thenar muscles is involved to some extent in
most of the gross movements of the thumb. The abductor
pollicis brevis contracts strongly during opposition and flexion
of the thumb as well as in abduction. The opponens shows
strong activity in abduction and flexion of the metacarpal, as
it does in opposition. The flexor pollicis brevis shows considerable activity in opposition as well as in flexion and in adduction. The adductor pollicis (which is, of course, not properly a
thenar muscle) is active in adduction and opposition, and to a
slight extent in flexion of the thumb.

Postures of Thumb

During extension produced by the extensors only the opponens pollicis and abductor pollicis brevis show reciprocal
activity (Forrest and Basmajian, 1965). During abduction, the
same two muscles show marked activity on the average
whereas the activity of the flexor pollicis brevis is slight. During flexion, the mean activity of the flexor pollicis brevis is
moderate to marked, but the opponens pollicis is only slightly
active and the abductor pollicis brevis is essentially inactive.

The occurrence of equal levels of activity in both the abductor pollicis brevis and the opponens pollicis during extension and abduction of the thumb cannot be rationalized
on the basis of their insertions. These are such that these
muscles would be expected to move the thumb in opposite

directions, especially during extension and to a lesser extent during abduction. Stabilization of the part in order to produce a smooth, even movement results from the significant activities of these muscles.

Not all thenar muscles are active during extension and flexion of the thumb. During flexion, the abductor pollicis brevis exhibits negligible activity; the opponens pollicis, slight activity on the average; and the flexor pollicis brevis, moderate-to-marked activity. Indeed, in the position of flexion, most subjects have little activity in both the opponens and abductor while the flexor is significantly active.

In one other position there is coincident activity and inactivity in the thenar muscles. During firm pinch between the thumb and the side of the flexed index finger (fig. 12.10),

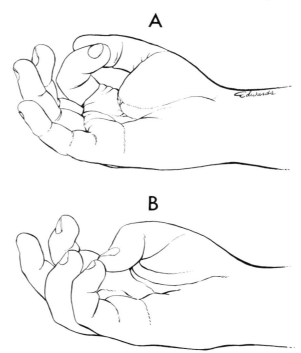

Fig. 12.10. A, Pinch between thumb and side of index finger—position 1 of figs. 12.11 and 12.12. B, Position 8.

only negligible activity is recorded from the abductor pollicis brevis (fig. 12.11). Yet the opponens pollicis and, in particular, the flexor pollicis brevis are significantly active.

Postures of Little Finger

During extension of the little finger, all three hypothenar muscles are rather inactive on the average. During abduction, although the abductor digiti minimi fulfils the function indicated by its name and is the dominant muscle, with strong activity, the other hypothenar muscles are also significantly active. During flexion, considerable activity occurs in all three hypothenar muscles.

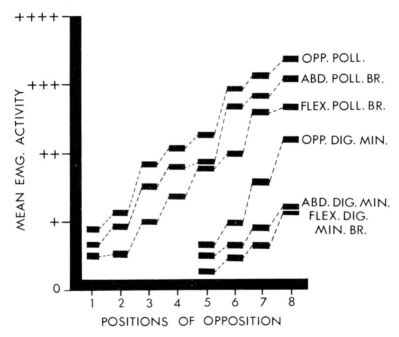

Fig. 12.11. Levels of EMG activity in six muscles with thumb opposition to fingers: 1 and 2, side and tip of index, and so on, to 7 and 8, side and tip of little finger (cf. fig. 12.10).

The abductor digiti minimi is very active during flexion of the little finger at the metacarpophalangeal joint. (The participation of this muscle in this position of the finger is also obvious by palpation.) Part of the explanation for this activity depends on the insertion of the muscle into the ulnar side of the base of the proximal phalanx. The abductor digiti minimi is also significantly active when the thumb is held opposed to either the ring or little finger (fig. 12.12). Some of this activity is possibly associated with the small degree of flexion at the fifth metacarpophalangeal joint that is required when the thumb and little finger are opposed. Yet such flexion is obviously not required during opposition of the thumb and ring finger. Some of the activity of the abduc-

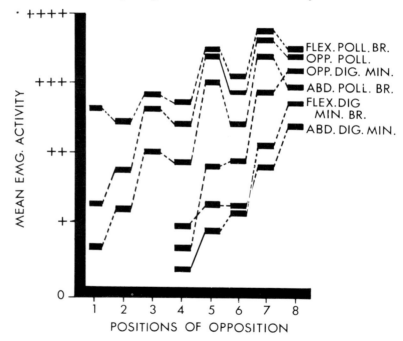

Fig. 12.12. Levels of EMG activity with firm pressure of thumb in same positions as in fig. 12.11.

tor digiti minimi, then, may be to provide stability, and simple abduction of the little finger may be the least important function of the abductor of this finger.

Positions of Opposition

During soft opposition of the thumb to the side or tip of each finger, the opponens is the most active of the thenar muscles and the flexor is the least active (fig. 12.11). The hypothenar muscles are recruited when the opposition is to the ring and little fingers. Then the opponens digiti minimi is the most active hypothenar muscle, but the thenar muscles are generally more active than the hypothenar muscles.

When opposition is firm the flexor pollicis brevis replaces the opponens pollicis as the dominant muscle, particularly in forceful opposition to the index and middle fingers. In forceful. opposition to the ring and little fingers, the activity of the opponens pollicis approaches and then equals that of the flexor pollicis brevis. During opposition to any finger the abductor pollicis brevis is the least active of the thenar muscles. With forceful opposition, higher levels of activity occur with firm opposition of the thumb to the side of any finger as compared with the activity during tip-to-tip opposition with the same finger (Forrest and Basmajian, 1965).

When the thumb is opposed firmly to the index and middle fingers, the flexor pollicis brevis replaces the opponens pollicis as the most active of the six muscles. The opponens, however, approaches and even equals the flexor in its activity during firm opposition to the ring and little fingers. Firm pinch between the thumb and the index and middle fingers is a grip position of day-to-day importance. The great power of the thumb, which enables this digit to balance the combined power of the fingers, has been attributed to the flexor pollicis brevis and to the mechanically advantageous position of the abductor pollicis.

As medial rotation of the first metacarpal is increased, the tendency of the head of the fifth metacarpal to be drawn in an anterolateral (volar-radial) direction is similarly increased.

The opponens digiti minimi is mainly responsible for this movement of the fifth metacarpal, and its action is almost reflexive in nature. The more active the opponens pollicis is in medially rotating the first metacarpal, the more active the opponens digiti minimi becomes. But the opponens pollicis is always the more active muscle. It is possible that beyond a certain degree of medial rotation of the first metacarpal, the two opponens muscles begin to act in unison to form the transverse metacarpal arch. Indeed, this might be expected when one views the two opponens muscles, with

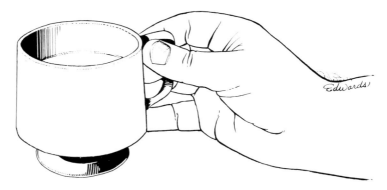

Fig. 12.13. Holding water-filled cup (*cf.* fig. 12.15).

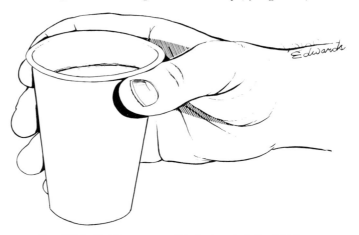

Fig. 12.14. Holding water-filled glass (*cf.* fig. 12.15).

the flexors retinaculum between, linking up the first and fifth metacarpal bones.

Thenar Muscles in Grip

The important rôle of the flexor pollicis brevis in firm grasp is illustrated in the positions of firmly clasping a dowel (or rounded handle) and of holding a cup of water (fig. 12.13). Although the flexor pollicis brevis is the most active muscle while the dowel is grasped firmly, this is not the case when a glass of water is also held firmly (fig. 12.14). Both the opponens pollicis and the abductor pollicis brevis are then more

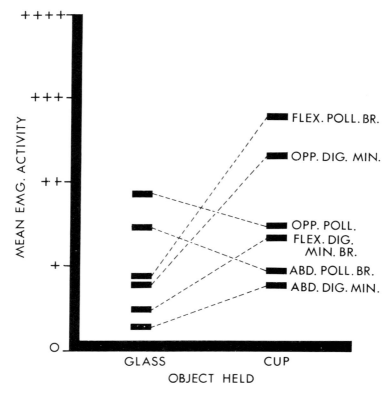

Fig. 12.15. Levels of EMG activity compared for six muscles while holding cup or glass of water.

active (fig. 12.15). Therefore, the more the thumb is abducted (as in holding the glass), the less the flexor brevis contributes to a firm grip. The activity of this muscle, which provides firmness of grip when only a small degree of abduction exists (as in holding the cup), is replaced by that of the opponens when a large amount of abduction is present. In the absence of significant flexor activity, this activity of the opponens coupled with that of the abductor provides the power of a firm grip.

In summary, not all thenar muscles are active in all thumb postures, but all hypothenar muscles are active in three basic postures of the little finger. Two somewhat different patterns of activity occur when the thumb is first softly and then firmly opposed to each of the fingers in a sequence that begins at the index and ends at the little finger. The flexor pollicis brevis is dominant in firm grip, particularly in grip between the thumb and two radial fingers, but a large degree of abduction of the thumb might possibly be a limiting factor in the activity of this muscle. The two opponens muscles seem to act as a unit in opposition of the thumb to both the ring and little fingers. Certain activity in some of the six muscles, which is inexplicable on a morphological basis, probably serves to provide stability.

Power Grip and Precision Handling

Taking the hand as a whole, in *power grip* the extrinsic muscles provide the major force, all of them being used in proportion to the force exerted (Long *et al.*, 1970). The major intrinsics of power grip are the interossei, used as phalangeal rotators and metacarpophalangeal flexors. The lumbricals are not significantly active. Except for hook grip, the thenar muscles are always recruited in power grip (see also p. 70 , Chapter 5).

In *precision handling* the extrinsics provide only gross reinforcement to the thenar muscles, adductor pollicis, the interossei and lumbricals. Long *et al.* (1970) point out that the interossei provide rotation to handled objects through abduction and adduction of the m-p joints. The lumbricals are not active when the interossei move objects towards the palm but they join their more powerful companions during translatory movements away from the palm.

Digital Musculature in Digito-Palmar Rubbing

Rubbing the palm of the hand by the pulps of all four fingers is a common enough operation, though usually an unconscious one. It is one of the actions of the fingers upon their possessor's own body; and it is *sufficient* (though not necessary) for explaining the muscular apparatus by which the three phalanges of a finger can be moved separately at their several joints.

Digito-palmar rubbing would seem to be a useful way for testing the actions of the various digital muscles clinically and for exercising them therapeutically. It has three advantages. First, it is directed towards a definite end, not merely a waving of fingers in the air. Secondly, it is easily demonstrated to the patient by a doctor or a physiotherapist. Thirdly, it can be practiced by the patient in the absence of either of these persons, and he or she has both a visual and a tactile gauge of the progress towards recovery of function being made.

Digito-palmar rubbing has two stages: an initial and a final. In one or other of the two stages of digito-palmar rubbing each of the digital muscles has a unique part to play, a part determined by a kinematic rather than by a kinetic end to be achieved by its action. Thus the flexor superficialis is not primarily an accessory to the flexor profundus in cases of rapid or forceful flexion of the middle phalanx, though this is its most frequent use. The independent flexion of this phalanx in the first stage of digito-palmar rubbing requires a muscle separate from the profundus.

Initial stage. The proximal and middle joints are fully flexed. The distal joints are fully extended, so that the pulp of each distal phalanx presses against the palm (minimus and anularis) or the thenar eminence (medius and index). In this stage the interossei and abductor-flexor mass of minimus flex the proximal joints, the extensor communis being therefore relaxed. The flexor superficialis flexes the middle joints. The lumbricals extend the distal joints. The proximal and distal joints are in their close-packed positions, the middle joints are not.

Final stage. This is the operational stage: throughout it the middle joints are kept flexed. The pulps of the fingers are made to slide distally along the palm and in firm contact with it, until they reach the skin over the heads of the metacarpals. This is done by an increasing flexion of the distal joints and an increasing extension of the proximal set. All joints are in loose-pack during this stage and the flexor profundus and the extensor communis are certainly active. The interossei relax, apparently at the start of the movement. This is easily verified for the 1st dorsal interosseus and the flexor-abductor mass of minimus by direct palpation.

Variant of initial stage. In this the pulps of the first three fingers are in contact with the thenar eminence alone; minimus is just to the ulnar side of it. This position involves an ulnar deviation of each proximal joint, together with (or followed by) a flexion at the same joint. These two movements in turn entail a third—a *conjunct rotation* of each finger in the sense of *supination.* This rotation is undone during the subsequent final stage.

The variant of the first phase clearly requires a flexor musculature for each proximal joint that consists of at least two parts, one of which is an ulnar deviator. The principle of parsimony would limit the total number to two, the other flexor element being a radial deviator; and we know that such pairs of muscles are present.

Finally, the extension of all four fingers after the second phase, followed by the hyperextension (dorsiflexion) of index and minimus, suggests that the latter two fingers have additional extensor muscles for their dorsiflexion, which is true. Thus the two forms of digito-palmar rubbing as we can see them suggest the presence of the complete set of digital muscles shown by dissection.

REFERENCES

Bäckdahl, M. and Carlsöö, S. (1961). Distribution of activity in muscles acting on the wrist (an electromyographic study). *Acta Morph. Neer.-Scandinav.*, *4:* 136-144.

Forrest, W.J. and Basmajian, J.V. (1965). Function of human thenar and hypothenar muscles: an electromyographic study of twenty-five hands. *J. Bone and Joint Surg.*, *47-A:* 1585-1594.

Long, C. (1968). Intrinsic-extrinsic muscle control of the fingers: electromyographic studies. *J. Bone and Joint Surg.*, *50-A:* 973-984.

Long, C., Conrad, P.W., Hall, E.W. and Furler, S.L. (1970). Intrinsic-extrinsic muscle control of the hand in power grip and precision handling. *J. Bone & Joint Surg.*, *52-A:* 853-867.

Person, R.S. and Roshtchina, N.A. (1958). Electromyographic investigation of coordinated activity of antagonistic muscles in movements of fingers of the human hand (Russian text). *J. Physiol. U.S.S.R.*, *94:* 455-462.

Tournay, A. and Paillard, J. (1953). Electromyographie des muscles radiaux a l'état normal. *Rev. Neurol.*, *89:* 277-279.

THIRTEEN

Hip, Thigh and Leg

GAIT

Although movements of the trunk and upper limbs also play a rôle in normal walking, the activity of the lower limbs evokes the greatest interest. A number of laboratories have devoted many years of study to the movements of the joints and accompanying muscular activity. In studies of gait, electromyography has been supplemented with other biomechanical techniques. Photographic methods, particularly high-frequency cinematography, have been used since the classic studies of Muybridge (1887). Photographic cyclograms, electronic accelerometers, recording of contacts of various parts of the foot with the ground, walking on force-plates (incorporating multiple, electronic, force- and displacement-transducers)—these and other techniques are now employed.

The six major determinants of human gait are (1) pelvic rotation, (2) pelvic tilt, (3) knee flexion, (4) hip flexion, (5) knee and ankle interaction and (6) lateral pelvic displacement (Saunders, Inman and Eberhart, 1953). Actually, the phenomenon of walking is much more complex, yet these are the components that provide the unifying principles. Locomotion is the translation of the centre of gravity through space along a path requiring the least expenditure of energy. Thus a pathological gait is an attempt to preserve as low a level of energy consumption as possible by exaggeration of the mo-

tions at the unaffected levels. When a person loses one determinant from the above six, compensation is reasonably effective. Loss of the determinant at the knee proves the most
costly. Loss of two determinants makes effective compensation
impossible; the cost in terms of energy consumption triples and
apparently discourages the patient to the point of his ad-
mitting defeat.

Conservation of Energy

Actually, normal human gait on a level surface at an average comfortable rate is extremely economic, and increases
the BMR only slightly above its level during standing or sitting. Greenlaw and Basmajian (1967-8; unpublished) showed
that all the muscles which act, generally do so at very low levels (see Basmajian, 1974). Thus, illustrations such as fig. 13.3
are deceptive; in that illustration the authors had to superim-
pose the results of many subjects to bring out the periodicity
of the action of the muscles, not the amount. When walking
is speeded beyond the "comfy cadence," both the bursts of
EMG activity (and thus the energy consumption) increase
sharply (Milner, Basmajian and Quanbury, 1971).

Phases in Walking Cycle

Traditionally, human gait is composed of two phases: (1)
stance, beginning when the heel strikes the ground, and (2)
swing, beginning with toeing-off (fig. 13.1). Fig. 13.2 illustrates
the interaction between the knee and ankle joints and the
phasic action of the major muscle groups. (The terms "knee
moment" and "ankle moment" refer to the action of muscles
about the knee or ankle which tend to change the angle of
these joints towards either flexion or extension.) Note the
following:

As the heel strikes the ground the hamstrings and pretibial muscles reach their peak of activity. Thereafter, the
quadriceps increases in activity as the torso is carried forward
over the limb, apparently in maintaining knee stability.

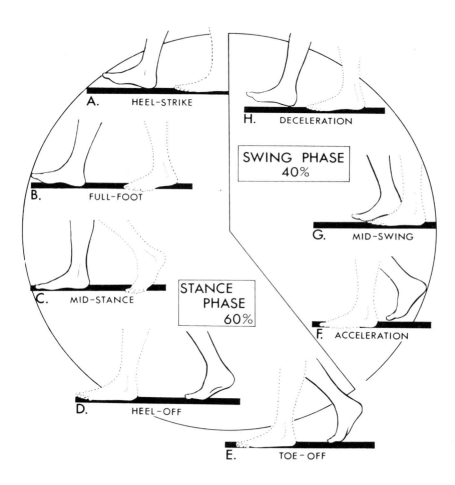

Fig. 13.1. A single walking cycle on a horizontal surface (60%—stance phase; 40%—swing phase). (After Gray and Basmajian, 1968.)

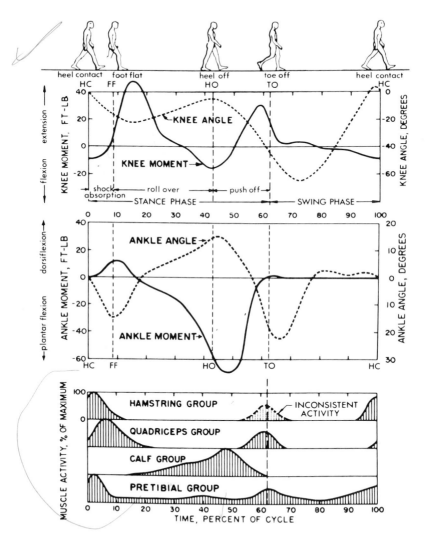

Fig. 13.2. Normal walking: knee and ankle moments (in foot-pounds) compared with muscular activity during one cycle of walking (right heel to right heel contact). (After Radcliffe, 1962.)

At heel-off the calf group of muscles build up a crescendo of activity which ceases with toe-off. This is the limit of the activity of the calf muscles, and it is the strong anti-gravity action needed at this moment. Before and during toe-off, quadriceps and sometimes the hamstrings reach another (but smaller) peak of activity.

The pretibial muscles maintain some activity all through the cycle, rising to a peak at heel-contact and to a smaller peak at toe-off.

During the stance phase the stabilizing function of the ankle plantar-flexors at the knee is most important (Radcliffe, 1962; Sutherland, 1966). The period of activity in the calf muscles and of knee extension and dorsiflexion of the foot correspond. Only at the end of plantar-flexion of the ankle does plantar-flexion of the foot occur. Knee extension occurs after quadriceps activity ceases; this is related to the fact that full extension of the knee never occurs during walking in the way that it does in standing (Murray et al., 1964).

Knee extension in the stance phase is brought about by the force of the plantar-flexors of the ankle resisting the dorsiflexion of the ankle; this dorsiflexion is in turn the resultant of extrinsic forces—kinetic forces, gravity and the reaction of the floor. Because the resultant of extrinsic forces proves to be dominant, increased dorsiflexion of the foot continues until heel-off begins. The restraining function of the ankle plantar-flexors in decelerating forward rotation of the tibia on the talus proves to be the key to their stabilizing action (Sutherland, 1966).

A movement of the torso and hip region that shifts their position over the feet initiates the movements of each foot during walking. Movements initiated in the trunk lead automatically to changes in the position of the leg and foot. Soleus stabilizes and adjusts the tibia on the talus. Apparently the movements of the ankle during walking occur as a reaction to muscular forces far removed from the foot. Inertial forces also play an important rôle throughout the lower limb.

A number of events occur during walking (fig. 13.3) which will be catalogued here for easy reference:

1. Contraction of the triceps surae is followed by that of gluteus maximus on the opposite side.

2. Contraction of the triceps surae corresponds to the first hump of the vertical accelerogram. However, it begins before the heel lifts off the ground and stops before the great toe leaves the ground.

3. Dorsiflexion of the foot begins at the time of maximum acceleration of the lower leg.

4. Tibialis anterior is usually biphasic in activity, but sometimes it is active for a short time after the foot is flat on the ground.

5. Contraction of iliopsoas occurs simultaneously with that of gluteus maximus of the opposite side.

6. Gluteus maximus shows activity at the end of the swing and at the beginning of the supporting phase. This is contrary to the general belief that its activity is not needed for ordinary walking. Perhaps gluteus maximus contracts to prevent or to control flexion at the hip joint.

7. Contraction of the gluteus maximus on the opposite side corresponds to the second hump of the vertical accelerogram.

8. Gluteus medius and gluteus minimus are active at the time that one would predict, i.e., during the supporting phase; however, some subjects show activity in the swing phase too.

9. Quadriceps femoris contracts as extension of the knee is being completed, not during the earlier part of extension when the action is probably a passive swing. Quadriceps continues to act during the early part of the supporting phase (when the knee is flexed and the centre of gravity falls behind it). Quadriceps activity occurs at the end of the supporting phase to

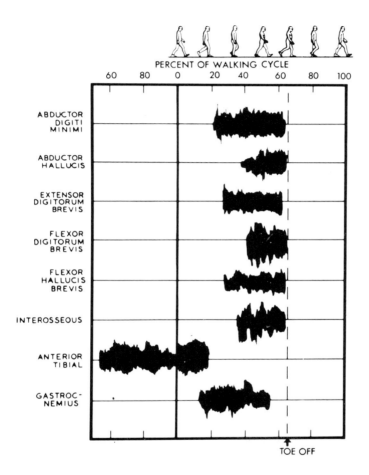

Fig. 13.3. Cycle of electromyographic activity during walking in muscles of the leg and foot. The apparently heavy activity is deceptive, resulting from superimposing of tracings from many subjects. (After Mann and Inman, 1964.)

fix the knee in extension, probably counteracting the tendency toward flexion imparted by gastrocnemius.

10. Extension of the knee begins at the time of maximum velocity of the leg.

11. In the supporting phase, activity occurs early in the calf muscles, hamstrings and gluteus maximus but ceases toward the end.

12. The hamstrings contract at the end of flexion and during the early extension of the thigh apparently to prevent flexion of the thigh before the heel is on the ground and to assist the movement of the body over the supporting limb. In some persons, the hamstrings also contract a second time in the cycle during the end of the supporting phase; this may prevent hip flexion.

13. In the swing phase, the hamstrings are inactive (even though knee flexion occurs).

HIP REGION AND THIGH

Iliopsoas

All textbooks agree that the muscle is obviously a flexor of the hip and probably has some influence on the lumbar vertebrae. It shows some slight activity during relaxed standing.

As one would expect, action potentials are recorded during flexion of the hip in almost any posture of the whole subject and in almost the whole range. The amount of activity varies directly with the effort or resistance. Marked activity appears in iliacus and psoas throughout flexion of the hip during "sit-up" from the "hook-lying" position, considerable activity occurring during the entire movement. Iliopsoas is quite active during extreme abduction of the hip and during lateral rotation. It is not a medial rotator. The only lumbar movement which consistently recruits psoas is a deliberate increase in lumbar lordosis while standing erect, but this is not dramatic (see Basmajian, 1974).

The Glutei and Tensor Fasciae Latae

Gluteus maximus is active only when heavy or moderate efforts are made in the movements classically ascribed to this muscle. It is active during extension of the thigh at the hip joint, lateral rotation, abduction against heavy resistance with the thigh flexed to 90° and adduction against resistance that holds the thigh abducted. Lateral rotation (but not the opposite) also produces activity in gluteus maximus.

While the whole muscle is engaged in extension and lateral rotation, only its upper part is abducent. As an abductor, gluteus maximus is a reserve source of power. It is not an important postural muscle even during forward swaying. In bending forwards it exhibits moderate activity. When straightening up from the toe-touching position it shows considerable activity throughout the movement.

The gluteus maximus is not a postural abductor muscle even when the subject is standing on one foot (as are the medius and minimus), but when the centre of gravity of the whole body is grossly shifted, activity of gluteus maximus occurs. In positions where one leg sustains most of the weight, the ipsilateral muscle is active in its upper or "abducent" part; apparently this is to prevent a drooping of the opposite side.

During standing, rotation of the trunk activates the muscle that is contralateral to the direction of rotation (i.e., corresponding to lateral rotation of the thigh). Forward bending at the hip joint and trunk recruits gluteus maximus, apparently to fix the pelvis.

Complete paralysis of gluteus maximus in no way disturbs ordinary walking even though the muscle shows phasic activity (p. 145).

GLUTEUS MEDIUS AND MINIMUS. The marked activity in the abductors when the subject stands on one foot is in sharp contrast with their quiescence during relaxed standing.

TENSOR FASCIAE LATAE. Duchenne clearly stated that the power of tensor fasciae latae as a rotator (in response to faradic stimulation) is weak, and we agree with this.

Adductors of the Hip Joint

Forming an enormous mass on the medial side of the upper thigh, the adductors must have considerable importance. In spite of this, their exact function was a matter of guesswork until recently.

The response of the adductors appears to be related to a postural response. Rather than being called upon as prime movers, they are facilitated through reflexes of the gait pattern. They are activated during movements of the knee, especially against resistance. But during movements of the hip, the rôle of the adductors is localized to their upper parts.

During free adduction, the adductor longus is always active while magnus is almost always silent unless resistance is offered. Both muscles are active during medial rotation but not during lateral rotation of the hip, settling a classic argument that usually supported the opposite view. The upper fibers of adductor magnus show the greatest activity.

During flexion of the thigh, the main activity occurs in the adductor longus, while the magnus is often completely silent. While standing in a relaxed natural posture, both muscles are inactive. However, weak activity sometimes appears when standing on one foot.

Hamstrings

The three hamstrings, biceps femoris, semimembranosus and semitendinosus, act on both hip joint and knee joint. The first is active in ordinary extension of the hip joint (in contrast to gluteus maximus which acts only against resistance) and in flexion and lateral rotation of the tibia at the knee. Biceps is active also in lateral rotation of the extended hip and in adduction against resistance of the abducted hip.

The semimembranosus and semitendinosus are active in extension and also during medial rotation of the hip, adduction against resistance of the abducted hip and flexion and medial rotation of the tibia at the knee joint. The hamstrings are quiescent in ordinary standing, but in flexion at the hip and in leaning forwards they are quite active as supporters against gravity.

It is not possible to forecast the exact phase of activity in a muscle during walking by only examining it while the limb is put through artificial tests of prime movers. For example, if semitendinosus and semimembranosus are examined while the two are producing a deliberate test movement, such as flexion of the knee, they are found to act synchronously. On the other hand, the semitendinosus flexes the knee during the swing phase of walking (on a treadmill) while semimembranosus acts mostly while the foot is on the ground. Although both heads of biceps femoris act synchronously during a free-moving test of flexion, the short head acts during the swing phase of walking while the long head acts as a stabilizer when the foot is on the ground. In general, the hamstrings are usually active during the transition from the swing phase to the stance phase.

There is now no doubt that the hamstrings do not act by regional contraction on only one joint. Studies of these muscles showed that the entire muscle contracts regardless of whether the upper or lower joint was moved. Which joint is to move as a consequence depends on the immobilization of the other joint by other agencies.

Rectus Femoris

The rectus femoris obviously is a flexor of the hip and extensor of the knee joint. Because flexion of the hip is closely associated with extension of the knee, one is not surprised to find a single muscle performing these two movements. As with the hamstrings, our studies on two-joint muscles demonstrated that normally the whole muscle contracts even with isolated movements of only one of the two joints. Rectus femoris also aids in abduction of the thigh, but it is relaxed in ordinary standing.

Gracilis and Sartorius

Though belonging to the adductor mass, the gracilis crosses and therefore acts on both hip and knee. It is active in flexion of the hip with the knee extended but is inactive if the knee is allowed to flex simultaneously. It adducts and rotates the femur medially (Jonsson and Steen, 1966). During flexion of the hip joint, gracilis is most active during the first part of flexion, both in free "basic movements" and during walking and cycling. In walking on a horizontal level and on a staircase its activity occurs during the swing phase. At the knee it is a flexor and medial rotator of the tibia, although in medial rotation and in relaxed standing its activity appears to be slight.

Sartorius is active during flexion of the thigh (regardless of whether the knee is straight or bent), during lateral rotation of the femur or abduction of the thigh and during flexion of the knee joint or medial rotation of the tibia. Both sartorius and gracilis may play a rôle in the fine postural adjustments of the hip and knee.

Vasti

The vasti, of course, are powerful extensors of the knee joint, but generally they are quiescent during relaxed standing, except when women wear high heels (Joseph and Nightingale, 1956).

During the movement of rising from the sitting to the standing position and vice versa, the activity in the three heads is not synchronized and equal. The vastus medialis is retarded and is not as active as the other two. In erect standing the activity

in the three heads falls rapidly. The three heads apparently
act in different ways in various phases of movement, but the
details remain obscure. There is a greater activity in vastus
medialis when the knee is held in extension with the hip joint
flexed or the knee joint (tibia) laterally rotated. On the other
hand, the vastus lateralis is more active in extension of the
knee when the hip is flexed or the knee joint (tibia) medially
rotated. During resisted extension of the knee, the various
parts of quadriceps come into action at different phases of the
movement (fig. 13.4).

Popliteus

Popliteus is a medial rotator of the tibia, its activity at the
start of flexion of the knee being related to the unlocking of
the knee joint. When a person stands in the semicrouched, knee-
bent position, continuous activity of the muscle occurs, because, when the knee is bent, the weight of the body tends to
slide the femur downward and forward on the slope of the tibia.

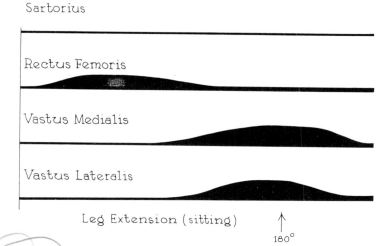

Fig. 13.4. Levels of muscular activity of rectus femoris and vasti compared during knee extension. (Sartorius, in contrast, remains inactive.)

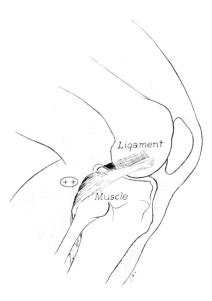

Fig. 13.5. Popliteus reinforces the anterior ligament in the knee-bent stance.

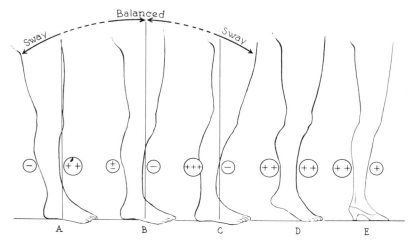

Fig. 13.6. Diagram of levels of muscular activity in the anterior and posterior muscles of the leg.

The continuous marked activity of popliteus aids the posterior cruciate ligament in preventing forward dislocation (fig. 13.5) (Barnett and Richardson, 1953).

Leg Muscles

Gastrocneumius is active intermittently in most persons during relaxed standing; very few women show no activity with high heels (fig. 13.6). The tibialis anterior and the peroneus longus (and, as we shall see, the intrinsic muscle of the foot) play no important active rôle in the normal static support of the long arches of the foot. Whatever postural activity there is in human legs during standing is intermittent.

Along with the peroneus longus, peroneus brevis acts only intermittently as a postural muscle, becoming very active in leaning forward and silent when leaning backward. Peroneal activity is pronounced during the propulsive phase of normal walking, and the activity of the two muscles is synchronous. Their discreteness suggests that each has its own special additional function(s).

REFERENCES

Barnett, C.H. and Richardson, A.T. (1953). The postural function of the popliteus muscle. *Ann. Phys. Med.*, 1: 177-179.

Basmajian, J.V. (1974). *Muscles Alive: their Functions Revealed by Electromyography*. Ed. 3. Williams & Wilkins Co., Baltimore.

Gray, E.G. and Basmajian, J.V. (1968). Electromyography and cinematography of leg and foot ("normal" and flat) during walking. *Anat. Rec.*, 161: 1-16.

Jonsson, B. and Steen, B. (1966). Function of the gracilis muscle. An electromyographic study. *Acta Morph. Neer.-Scandinav.*, 6: 325-341.

Joseph, J. and Nightingale, A. (1956). Electromyography of muscles of posture: leg and thigh muscles in women, including the effects of high heels. *J. Physiol.*, 132: 465-468.

Mann, R. and Inman, V.T. (1964). Phasic activity of intrinsic muscles of the foot. *J. Bone and Joint Surg.*, 46-A: 469-481.

Milner, M., Basmajian, J.V. and Quanbury, A.O. (1971). Multifactorial analysis of walking by electromyography and computer. *Am. J. Phys. Med.*, 50: 235-258.

Murray, P.M., Drought, A.B. and Kory, R.C. (1964). Walking patterns of normal men. *J. Bone and Joint Surg.*, *46-A:* 335-360.

Muybridge, E. (1887). *The Human Figure in Motion.* Reprinted in 1955 by Dover Publications, Inc., New York.

Radcliffe, C.W. (1962). The biomechanics of below-knee prostheses in normal, level, bipedal walking. *Artif. Limbs.*, *6:* 16-24.

Saunders, J.B. deC.M., Inman, V.T. and Eberhart, H.D. (1953). The major determinants in normal and pathological gait. *J. Bone and Joint Surg.*, *35-A:* 543-558.

Sutherland, D.H. (1966). An electromyographic study of the plantar flexors of the ankle in normal walking on the level. *J. Bone and Joint Surg.*, *48-A:* 66-71.

FOURTEEN

Foot and Ankle

In spite of substantial research over the past fifty years, a clear understanding of the functional anatomy of the foot remains elusive. Various studies have provided information on its static functions, but such information is incomplete because the foot is also a dynamic structure. Even the old theory that the arches of the foot—as arches—are of vital significance calls for re-examination.

Acceptable definitions of a "normal" and a flat foot do not exist, with dictionaries lamely defining flat foot as "a condition in which one or more of the arches of the foot have flattened out". Most descriptions of a "normal" foot suggest an idealized structure with lateral and medial longitudinal arches and a transverse arch, the last supposedly crossing the heads of the five metatarsals.

The fact is that the notion of medial and transverse arches arose from an attempt to describe the foot in terms of engineering structures already known, from a confusion between something curved (arcuate) and a true arch. As was shown in Chapter 8, the foot, excluding the toes, is a twisted plate the most anterior and posterior parts of which are in full contact with the ground (through the skin) in the standing position. It is this twist which generates the so-called medial and transverse arches (fig. 14.1). The whole osteo-ligamentous plate has a basic longitudinal curvature imposed upon it by the true arch of the foot, that part whose posterior pillar is the upwardly sloping

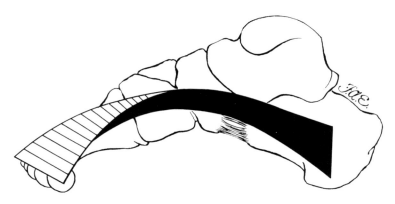

Fig. 14.1. The "twisted plate" which generates the medial arch. In this scheme, the toes (which bear no weight) are removed.

calcaneus, whose keystone is the cuboid bone and whose anterior pillar is composed of the fifth and fourth metatarsals. One can talk of a flat foot only if this arch be flattened. The height of the medial "arch" will be greater when the foot is twisted, that is, when the feet are side-by-side on the ground—greatest when the feet are crossed in a standing subject. It will be least when the feet are abducted and will then approximate to that of the true arch. Moreover, the possible increase in height of the medial "arch" will always be less in those with long feet than those with short feet since the twisting of the foot-plate will be distributed over a greater length, as is the case with many Africans and many Europeans.

It will, no doubt, take some time before this concept leads to a recasting of the language used about feet by both anatomists and clinicians, even though it is easily verified both in the dissecting room and by radiology. In particular, it will have to be realised that a patient may not have a "flat foot" even when a medial arch is not very evident, and also that there is no necessary association between a painful foot and a flat foot, as Jones (1944) and later Perkins (1947) have warned us. Lastly, there is no point in asking whether a medial arch is or is not beneficial. It is simply a necessary consequence of a twistable foot such as men have. This, however, is a necessity for true bipedal standing of the human type.

"Toe-out" and "toe-in", which describe the angle made by the feet in reference to the line or path of walking, have given similar concern in the past. In a long series of subjects, Morton (1952) found that the average toe-out during walking was 7.5°. Because a flatfooted person often toes out markedly in his walking, some clinicians maintain that it is an "inefficient" manner of walking, but others suggest that excessive toe-out may have some purpose and therefore question the rationale of efforts to "correct" it.

Arch Supporting Mechanisms

After extended study, Hicks (1961) described three different, interdependent supporting mechanisms: a "beam", a "truss" and a "muscle mechanism". Experiments with leg-and-foot preparations from cadavers established that strong ligaments in the sole of the foot uniting neighbouring bones make the foot behave like a solid curved beam (fig. 14.1). The "truss" theory proposes that the plantar aponeurosis acts as a tie to prevent separation of the two ends of the arch. Further, through a windlass effect, the plantar aponeurosis is tensed by passive dorsiflexion of the great toe (fig. 14.2). Apparently this mechanism provides an adjustable arch during walking, especially when the heel is raised off the ground and the body weight shifts onto the ball of the foot. Finally, the "muscle mechanism" stabilizes a constantly changing position of the line of weight of the body while standing.

Muscular Function in the Foot

Keith (1929) formulated the theory that muscles actively hold up the arches; otherwise a flat foot would result. This theory, based on extensive phylogenetic evidence, received support from Willis (1935) who concluded from tension experiments in cadavers that the tibialis posterior and peroneus

A.

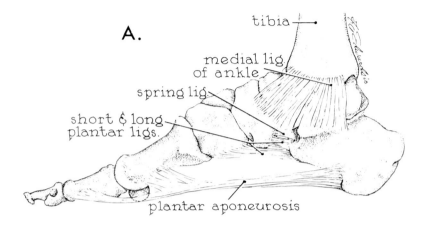

tibia

medial lig.
of ankle

spring lig.

short & long
plantar ligs.

plantar aponeurosis

B.

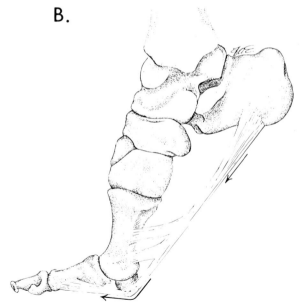

Fig. 14.2. A, Plantar ligaments which help support the arch of the static
foot. B, The windlass effect that tightens the plantar aponeurosis.

longus muscles keep the medial arch from collapsing. He claimed that the tibialis posterior maintained the normal relationship of the navicular and talus near the summit of the medial arch and so prevented distortion of the front part of the foot in a lateral direction, *i.e.*, an abducted forefoot.

Other investigators disagreed with Keith's theory, again on indirect evidence, largely the evolutionary changes in the foot. Emphasizing the firmness of bones and the strength of ligaments, R. L. Jones (1941) found that the tibialis posterior and peroneal muscles can support only 15 to 20% of the body weight. In addition, Harris and Beath (1948) concluded from an extensive survey that a balance exists between the ligaments in the sole and the active contraction of muscles in both leg and foot. They placed greater importance on the ligaments, but thought the muscles would be quick to respond if the ligaments failed. They defined a stable foot as one which has interlocking articular processes at joints that are firmly joined by ligaments, and a less stable foot as one that needs muscular support because it lacks ligamentous support. Independently, F. Wood Jones (1944) had also concluded that there is an equilibrium between the passive ligaments and the active muscles in support of the arches of the foot, fallen arches resulting if this balance were upset. However, he believed that all the muscles, both intrinsic and extrinsic, are in a steady state of partial contraction.

This was the confused state of affairs until electromyography became available. We found that the tibialis anterior, peroneus longus and intrinsic muscles of the foot take no part in support of the arches during standing, regardless of any rôle they may have during locomotion (Basmajian and Bentzon, 1954). Smith (1954) reported that, although the anterior, posterior and peroneal muscles of the leg were inactive in a standing position, they were active while walking. Later, we showed in a study of six leg and foot muscles with extremely heavy loads (up to 400 pounds) applied at the knee of seated subjects that muscles are not significant in providing static support. How-

ever, the muscles do provide a dynamic reserve, especially
during the take-off phase of walking.

While some investigators report that the anterior leg muscles are active throughout the walking cycle, with peak activity at heel-strike and again when the foot leaves the ground,
others have found that the anterior crural muscles are active
during walking only while the foot is off the ground. Most
agree that the posterior muscles are active while the foot is
on the ground.

Mann and Inman (1964), in their study of phasic activity,
showed that the actions of the intrinsic muscles are related to
the axes of the subtalar and transverse tarsal joints of the foot
(fig. 14.3). They believed that the intrinsic muscles stabilize
the joints, *i.e.*, the foot may act at times as if it did not have
any joints. Flatfooted subjects require more activity of the

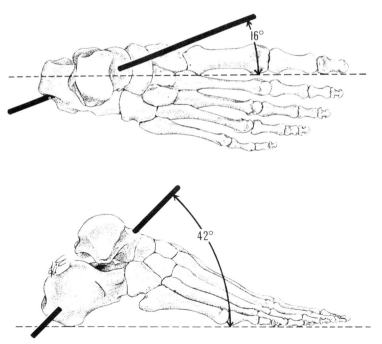

Fig. 14.3. Axis of the subtalar joint (modified, after Mann and Inman).

muscles, apparently to hold the joints of the foot in a rigid position, but the intrinsic muscles are not needed in the standing position.

This state of confusion led us to undertake a detailed electromyographic study of leg and foot muscles in normal and flat-footed subjects (Gray and Basmajian, 1968). The details have been reported elsewhere; here we shall consider the main findings and conclusions.

DEFINITIONS OF THE WALKING CYCLE. Walking forward, in effect, is a process of losing and regaining body balance. A "gait cycle" is the period from the time one of the feet strikes the ground until the same foot makes contact with the ground again (fig. 14.4). The gait cycle has two subdivisions, the "stance" and the "swing" phases.

The *stance phase* is when the foot is on the ground. It is divided into "heel-strike", "full-foot", "mid-stance", "heel-off" and finally "toe-off". At the point of "mid-stance" in the cycle the body weight is entirely over the foot.

The *swing phase* is divided into three parts: "acceleration", "mid-swing" and "deceleration" (fig. 13.1). At the moment of acceleration the leg is behind the trunk; at mid-swing, directly under; and at deceleration, well in front, ready to make contact with the ground at heel-strike.

About 60% of a gait cycle is occupied by the stance phase and 40% by the swing phase, the speed of walking governing the time each leg will remain in contact with the ground. There is a time at the beginning and at the end of each cycle when both feet are on the ground. These times are prolonged at slower speeds.

LEVEL WALKING: ACCUSTOMED FOOT POSITION

Tibialis Anterior

This muscle has been a favored object of attention, and so it is commonly accepted that peak EMG activity occurs in it at heel-strike of the stance phase. Our movies show the foot to be inverted and dorsiflexed at this time.

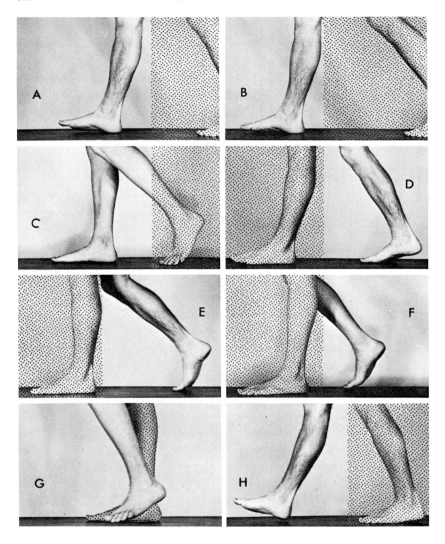

Fig. 14.4. Photographs of normal and flatfooted subjects to show special features of the right foot (except in frame G) during the walking cycle. A, heel-strike (sole of normal forefoot turned medially); B, full-foot (normal, lateral border and heel making contact); C, mid-stance (flat foot, in neutral position); D, heel-off (normal, heel turned medially); E, toe-off (normal); F, acceleration (flat foot); G, mid-swing of LEFT flat foot; H, deceleration (sole of right normal forefoot turned medially).

Notwithstanding the above, there has been no general agreement as to the function of tibialis anterior at heel-strike. Without offering direct evidence, some suggest only that it counteracts forces applied to the heel by the ground, while others propose that the tibialis anterior decelerates the foot at heel-strike and lowers it to the ground by gradual lengthening (eccentric contraction). Perhaps the clinical condition known as "drop-foot" due to paralysis of the tibialis anterior forces this conclusion.

During the more central moments of the stance phase (full-foot, mid-stance and heel-off) modern techniques reveal no tibialis anterior activity in "normal" subjects. Our flatfooted subjects and those of Battye and Joseph (1966) are like the "normals" except for extended activity into full-foot. Curiously, the movies of our flatfooted subjects show the foot staying inverted during full-foot, maintaining inversion in order to distribute the body weight along its lateral border.

A peak of EMG activity that occurs at toe-off of the stance phase is apparently related to dorsiflexion of the ankle, presumably to permit the toes to clear the floor.

Although earlier workers believed that there is a slight fall in the activity of tibialis anterior at mid-swing, there is, in fact, a period of electrical *silence* at mid-swing. The explanation emerges from our movies which show the foot everting at the end of "acceleration" and remaining everted through mid-swing. This allows for adequate clearance, while the inactivity of the invertor fits the concept of reciprocal inhibition of antagonists. We conclude that the brief period of electrical silence of tibialis anterior is essential.

The peak of activity at toe-off tapers to a slight-to-moderate level of activity during acceleration of the swing phase. Conversely, prior activity in deceleration of the swing phase builds up to a peak of activity at heel-strike. Thus, the pattern of activity of tibialis anterior is biphasic. Apparently, tibialis anterior is in part responsible for dorsiflexion during acceleration and for inversion of the foot during deceleration of the swing phase.

The pattern of activity of tibialis anterior suggests that it does not lend itself to direct support of the arches during walking. At heel-strike, when the muscle shows its greatest activity, the pressure of body weight is negligible. Conversely, during maximum weight-bearing at mid-stance when all the body weight is balanced on one foot, the tibialis anterior is silent. When the activity resumes at toe-off, the weightbearing of the involved foot is minimal.

Tibialis Posterior

During ordinary walking tibialis posterior shows activity at mid-stance of the stance phase. The movies show the foot remaining inverted throughout full-foot and turning to a neutral position (between inversion and eversion) just before mid-stance. First, the fourth and fifth metatarsal heads make contact; then, as the foot everts increasingly toward neutral, more of the ball of the foot makes contact at mid-stance until the entire contact-area of the foot is applied. Although the tibialis posterior is an invertor in non-weightbearing movements of the foot, its rôle at "mid-stance" appears to be a restraining one to prevent the foot from everting past the neutral position.

R. L. Jones (1941, 1945) showed in human cadaveric preparations that the tibialis posterior distributes body weight among the heads of the metatarsals. In living subjects he showed that a lateral torque on the tibia results in an increase or shift of body weight onto all but the first metatarsal head; a medial torque has the opposite effect. He concluded that by inverting the instep of the foot the tibialis posterior increases the proportion of body weight borne by the lateral side of the foot. Sutherland (1966) concluded that the plantar flexors, including the tibialis posterior, have a restraining function, to control or decelerate medial rotation of the leg and thigh observed at mid-stance; by controlling the eversion of the foot at mid-stance, the tibialis posterior provides an appropriate placement of the foot. In our flatfooted subjects, the EMG activity of tibialis posterior in the early stance phase is consistent with the maintenance of an inverted position during full-foot. By maintaining inversion the foot is supported in order to keep the body weight on the lateral border of the sole.

The foot must be inverted to accomplish lateral weight-bearing in the early "moments" of the stance phase. This of course is because the middle part of the medial border of the foot does not bear body weight in "normal" subjects; the lateral border with its strong plantar ligaments is well equipped to bear the stresses of body weight in walking (Napier, 1957).

Although tibialis posterior is often considered to be a plantarflexor of the ankle, during level walking with an accustomed foot position it shows *nil* activity at heel-off (when plantarflexion of the ankle takes place to raise the heel) (fig. 14.5). (This is not to deny that tibialis posterior may be a plantarflexor of the ankle when more powerful contractions are needed.)

Flexor Hallucis Longus

At mid-stance, when the entire body weight is concentrated on one foot, flexor hallucis longus shows its greatest activity. Flexing the big toe apparently positions and stabilizes it during mid-stance. During heel-off, our movies show the big toe hyperextended. Although Napier (1957) felt that the flexor hallucis longus helps maintain overall balance and prevents instability induced by excessive extension of the big toe, our EMG observations support this only for the flatfooted subjects and then only weakly. There is a slight activity during heel-off which may be related to preventing overextension and so giving a better balance. In contrast, the "normal" subjects show negligible activity. Consequently, one may conclude that the flexor hallucis longus is not needed in most "normal" subjects to play this rôle.

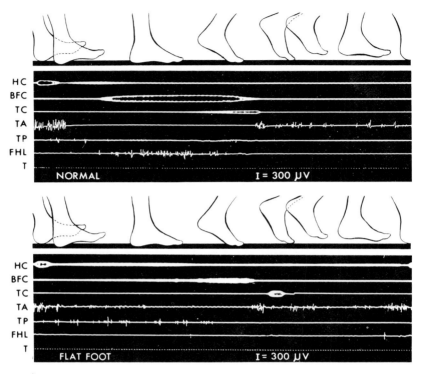

Fig. 14.5. EMGs of tibialis anterior (TA), tibialis posterior (TP) and flexor hallucis longus (FHL) during level walking with an accustomed foot position in "normal" (upper set) and flatfooted (lower set) subjects. Diagrams of foot positions are generalized; the exact positions are indicated by records of heel contact (HC), ball of foot contact (BFC) and toe contact (TC). Time marker (T): 10 ms. intervals.

Peroneus Longus

The pattern of activity of the peroneus longus confirms the findings of many who have suggested that the peroneus longus helps to stabilize the leg and foot during mid-stance. Our movies and electromyograms show how the peroneus longus and tibialis posterior, working in concert, control the shift from inversion during full-foot to neutral at mid-stance. Thus the opinion of R. L. Jones is again confirmed; from static studies, he inferred that peroneus longus is related to eversion of the foot at mid-stance during level walking. Sutherland further concluded that peroneus longus, like tibialis posterior, is involved in controlling rotatory movements at the ankle and foot. We found that eversion of the foot and medial rotation of the lower limb occur together. One may conclude that the peroneus longus is in part responsible for returning the foot to, and maintaining it in, a neutral position at mid-stance.

Throughout most of the stance phase, peroneus longus is generally more active in flatfooted subjects than in "normal" subjects. This appears to be a compensatory mechanism called forth by faulty architecture.

During heel-off, our movies showed some inversion while peroneus longus, an evertor, is active, and the invertors are relaxed. Duchenne (1867) first suggested that the inversion is caused by triceps surae. We believe the activity in peroneus longus affords stability by preventing excessive inversion, thus maintaining appropriate contact with the ground.

In flatfooted subjects, the interplay of activity between peroneus longus and tibialis posterior appears to play a special rôle in stabilizing the foot during mid-stance and heel-off. At mid-stance the tibialis posterior is notably more active, but at heel-off the emphasis shifts to peroneus longus.

Abductor Hallucis and Flexor Digitorum Brevis

These two muscles become active at mid-stance and continue through to toe-off in "normal" subjects; in flatfooted subjects most show activity from heel-strike to toe-off. Perhaps the flexor digitorum brevis and abductor try to grip the ground since they are flexors of the toes. Although others are not opposed to this idea, they believe that the muscles are also in an ideal location to help support the arches. Our findings tend to confirm this opinion only for flatfooted subjects because they showed higher mean levels of muscular activity.

TOE-OUT AND TOE-IN FOOT POSITION (LEVEL WALKING)

A parallel position of the feet during walking has been advocated by some physicians and physical educators for therapeutic reasons and by others for esthetic reasons. What is the correct position of the feet during walking? Actually, most individuals toe out slightly (at an angle of 7.5°), but some walk with the feet in a toe-in position. An exaggerated toe-out position affects the mean levels of activity more than toe-in does. Nevertheless, the muscles retain their basic pattern of activity seen with the accustomed foot position. The notable changes in mean levels of activity—some are increases, some decreases —occur in the early part of the stance phase.

The toe-out or toe-in position determines the manner in which the heel strikes the ground at the beginning of the stance phase. When one walks with the feet pointed straight ahead the heel strikes the ground near its midline, but the toe-out position of 45° places the extreme lateral edge of the heel on the ground first. Conversely, the medial side of the heel strikes the ground first when walking with the foot in the toe-in position.

Although the toe-out position is manifested in the foot, it is chiefly the result of lateral rotation of the hip joint. With the toe-out position the lateral border of the foot is effectively placed on the ground from the very onset of the stance phase. Whilst one might guess that muscles which can invert the foot (and so set it on its lateral border) should show less activity at full-foot, yet they generally show higher activity (e.g., tibialis anterior). This must be because they are in a better position to lower the foot to the ground in the toe-out position.

At heel-off, the increased activity of flexor hallucis longus is consistent with that expected from pressure studies (Elftman, 1934). Pressure from body weight during toe-out walking is concentrated on the first metatarsal of the big toe. However, with the accustomed foot position, the pressure is distributed better across the five metatarsal heads. Thus the flexor hallucis longus should be more active in maintaining balance at heel-off during toe-out walking.

The toe-in position is also mainly the result of rotation at the hip joint and not in the foot. Walking with the foot in the toe-in position generally shows lesser changes in the levels of muscular activity than in the toe-out position when both are compared with the accustomed position. However, some of the activity in the toe-in position may be due to inversion resulting from the effort of keeping the foot in a toe-in position.

In flatfooted subjects, levels of muscular activity are generally less affected by walking in the exaggerated toe-out or toe-in positions than is the case for the accustomed foot position. Harris and Beath (1948) thought that flatfooted individuals had a greater degree of movement between the bones of the foot than "normal" individuals, and Close (1964) confirmed their opinion. He found a greater freedom of movement in the joints while walking, especially in the subtalar joint, when compared to "normal" subjects. Perhaps the greater freedom of movement in the bones allows the flatfooted subjects to assume the toe-out and toe-in position more easily while the relationship of bones is retained.

The toe-out and toe-in foot positions during walking affect the levels of muscular activity in various ways when compared with the accustomed foot position, but it does not necessarily follow that one foot position is more advantageous than another during walking. Indeed, the position of the foot during walking is an individual characteristic.

WALKING UP AND DOWN AN INCLINE

Muscle action is not the only factor which determines the movement of the body while walking. Amongst others, the force of gravity and a purposeful loss of body balance are influential. Even in walking downhill at 5.5° or more, the force of gravity is not an aid but a handicap; additional effort is

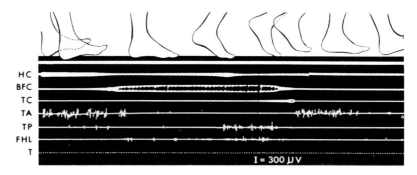

Fig. 14.6. EMGs of tibialis anterior (TA), tibialis posterior (TP) and flexor hallucis longus (FHL) during walking up an incline (with an accustomed foot position) in a "normal" subject. Diagrams of foot positions are generalized; the exact positions are indicated by records of heel contact (HC), ball of foot contact (BFC) and toe contact (TC). Time marker (T): 10 ms. intervals.

required to overcome the reverse effect of gravity. We found that some muscles show obvious changes.

Walking up an incline (fig. 14.6) modifies the manner in which the foot strikes the ground. Rather than the usual type of heel-strike found in level walking, the foot is practically "placed" on the ground. Dorsiflexion and inversion of the foot are superfluous in this modified placement of the foot, and therefore tibialis anterior shows correspondingly less activity.

The increased activity of tibialis anterior at full-foot and mid-stance may be related to maintaining the position of the leg so that the body can be balanced over the leg and foot by mid-stance. The tibialis anterior of subjects standing on an incline is active to keep the leg poised over the foot as a base of support. Thus, although the tibialis anterior acts on the foot when only a part of the foot is on the ground, it may be acting on the leg when the sole of the foot is on the ground.

The tibialis posterior showed activity at heel-off in about half of our subjects; here the tibialis posterior is probably acting as a plantarflexor in response to the additional muscular effort needed to walk up an incline. It has been suggested that if one leans farther forward to create a further imbalance of the body when walking up an incline less effort from the muscles is needed. Perhaps those subjects who show *nil* activity unconsciously make use of this change of body position.

Some subjects show activity in peroneus longus during the swing phase when walking up an incline. When compared to level ground, the inclined surface offers an additional obstacle. Although it would be possible for the foot to clear the floor by greater flexion of the more proximal joints (such as the knee and hip), nevertheless, the foot everts; apparently this provides a smoother and more efficient gait.

One would expect some changes in levels of activity in muscles of the lower limb when walking down an incline, since gravity is now acting positively on the body. Indeed all the muscles (with the exception of tibialis anterior) generally show lower mean levels when compared to level walking. It appears that gravity has made the performance of walking easier as far as movements and muscular activity of the foot are concerned. One may argue that perhaps these changes are due to a modified placement of the foot, but our movies do not confirm this, showing the foot making similar movements in both level walking and walking down our incline.

The acceleration due to gravity increases the walking speed. This suggests that some muscles are necessary to control the descent down the incline. In the early stance phase the tibialis anterior may help to resist excessive walking speeds.

GENERAL CONSIDERATIONS

The tibiales anterior and posterior, flexor hallucis longus, peroneus longus, abductor hallucis and flexor digitorum brevis are all concerned with both movements and restraints in the foot during walking. The inversion of the foot seen at heel-strike appears to be related primarily to the activity of tibialis anterior, although tibialis posterior, abductor hallucis and flexor digitorum brevis show slight mean activity in flatfooted subjects. All except flexor hallucis longus may be attempting to maintain inversion in flatfooted subjects during full-foot. However, maintenance of inversion in most "normal" subjects may be due to factors not yet studied.

Dorsiflexion and inversion, which occur at acceleration and deceleration, respectively, are in part related to the action of tibialis anterior during the swing phase. However, none of the muscles studied could be credited with producing the movement of eversion that occurs at about mid-swing.

During toe-in and toe-out walking or when the floor is inclined or declined, the muscles respond to these conditions whilst retaining their basic pattern seen in ordinary level walking. Indeed, these modes of walking have served as a test for the validity of the patterns of activity seen in level walking with the accustomed foot position. They also show that the muscles respond individually to situations where the demands upon them differ.

ARCH SUPPORT

The most controversial function of the muscles that traverse the foot is the support of the arches. Our observations on the flatfooted subjects confirm the opinions of Harris and Beath regarding what we would call the contingent support of the foot by muscles. They thought that a flatfooted person needs active muscular support during walking, and our flatfooted subjects show statistically significant differences from "normal" subjects in mean activity early in the stance phase. Moreover, the slightly higher mean levels of muscular activity generally seen in these subjects suggest that they may be actively supporting the arches of the foot. It appears, then, that besides providing movements of the joints of the foot, propulsion of body and stability of joints as in "normal" subjects during walking, the muscles of flatfooted subjects may also help to support (or attempt to support) the arches of the foot during locomotion.

REFERENCES

Basmajian, J. V. and Bentzon, J. W. (1954). An electromyographic study of certain muscles of the leg and foot in the standing position. *Surg. Gynec. and Obst.*, *98:* 662–66.

Battye, C. K. and Joseph, J. (1966). An investigation by telemetering of the activity of some muscles in walking. *Med. and Biol. Eng.*, *4:* 125–135.

Close, J. R. (1964). *Motor Function in the Lower Extremity: Analyses by Electronic Instrumentation.* Charles C Thomas, Springfield, Ill.

Duchenne, G. B. A. (1867). *Physiologie des mouvements.* Transl. by E. B. Kaplan (1949), W. B. Saunders, Philadelphia and London.

Elftman, H. (1934). A cinematic study of the distribution of pressure in the human foot. *Anat. Rec.*, *59:* 481–491.

Gray, E. G. and Basmajian, J. V. (1968). Electromyography and cinematography of leg and foot ("normal" and flat) during walking. *Anat. Rec.*, *161:* 1–15.

Harris, R. I. and Beath, T. (1948). Hypermobile flat-foot with short tendo achillis. *J. Bone and Joint Surg.*, *30-A:* 116–140.

Hicks, J. H. (1961). The three weight bearing mechanisms of the foot. In *Biomechanical Studies of the Musculo-Skeletal System.* Edited by F. G. Evans. Charles C Thomas, Springfield, Ill.

Jones, F. W. (1944). *Structure and Function as Seen in the Foot.* Baillière, Tindall and Cox, London.

Jones, R. L. (1941). The human foot. An experimental study of its mechanics, and the role of its muscle and ligaments in the support of the arch. *Am. J. Anat.*, *68:* 1–39.

Jones, R. L. (1945). The functional significance of the declination of the axis of the subtalar joint. *Anat. Rec.*, *93:* 151–159.

Keith, A. (1929). The history of the human foot and its bearing on orthopaedic practice. *J. Bone and Joint Surg.*, *11:* 10–32.

Mann, R. and Inman, V. T. (1964). Phasic activity of intrinsic muscles of the foot. *J. Bone and Joint Surg.*, *46-A:* 469–481.

Morton, D. J. (1952). *Human Locomotion and Body Form.* Williams & Wilkins Co., Baltimore.

Napier, J. R. (1957). The foot and the shoe. *Physiotherapy*, *43:* 65–74.

Perkins, G. (1947). Pes planus or instability of the longitudinal arch. *Proc. Roy. Soc. Med.*, *41:* 31–40.

Smith, J. W. (1954). Muscular control of the arches of the foot in standing. *J. Anat.*, *88:* 152–163.

Sutherland, D. H. (1966). An electromyographic study of the plantar flexors of the ankle in normal walking on the level. *J. Bone and Joint Surg.*, *48-A:* 66–71.

Willis, T. A. (1935). Function of the long plantar muscles. *Surg. Gynec. and Obst.*, *60:* 150–156.

FIFTEEN

Head and Neck

This chapter deals briefly with complex and often obscure movements of profound significance to life. Though not the concern of the routine textbooks of kinesiology aimed at college students, these functions are nevertheless controlled by muscles and so we cannot ignore them here. Indeed some of the most interesting mechanisms of biological movement are exemplified in this area.

Certain omissions have been made, *e.g.*, muscles of facial expression, middle ear, palate, pharynx and larynx. The reasons are twofold: first, these muscles are very specialized; and, second, little kinesiologic electromyography has been done in these areas as yet.

Cervical and Atlanto-occipital Movements

In Chapter 9, we discussed the vertebral column as a whole. Here our concern is with the localized posture and movements of the head and neck insofar as they have been revealed by scientific studies that go beyond the well established anatomy of the region.

The structure of the cervical vertebrae allows a freedom of motion denied the other vertebral regions. Thus flexion and extension, lateral flexion, and rotation are produced by the many muscles running from the trunk to the skull and vertebrae, from vertebra to vertebra and from cervical vertebrae to the skull. Much of this motion occurs in the atlanto-occipital and atlanto-axial joints, but isolated motion at these joints probably occurs only rarely except in slight head-shaking and nodding movements where a conscious effort is made to localize the movement. In such cases a complex organization is called on by the nervous system to inhibit certain muscles that normally would act reflexly and to contract others to stabilize vertebrae which otherwise would also move.

The fundamental anatomy of the dens and its ligaments and of the transverse ligament of the atlas are too well described in textbooks to be rehearsed here (fig. 15.1). The pivotal movement of the dens within its osseofibrous collar is limited by the simultaneous tightening of the two alar ligaments (fig. 117). No EMG studies of the muscles that act locally on these joints have been reported, but it is safe to assume that the various short muscles surrounding the region contribute heavily to the movement. These include the recti capitis (anterior, lateral, posterior minor and major) and the obliques (superior and inferior). Yet it is difficult to limit the motive power of the joints to these muscles alone, for there are many other muscles which span them and which certainly come into

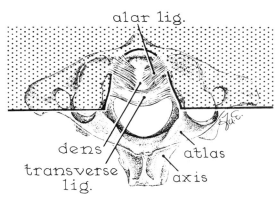

Fig. 15.1. The alar ligaments and dens of the axis viewed from above. (The dotted area represents a portion of the occipital bone to indicate location of foramen magnum.)

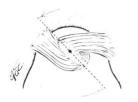 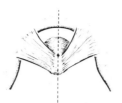 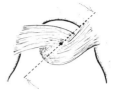

Fig. 15.2. Pivoting of the dens in either direction is limited by both alar ligaments ("check" ligaments).

play whenever powerful torsion or bending movements are required. These include the sterno(cleido)mastoid, scalenes, longus colli, longissimus, splenius, semispinalis and various intrinsic small muscles. Unfortunately only a few of these have been studied electromyographically to the extent that new ideas have emerged concerning their influence on the spine.

Longus colli and longissimus are almost completely inactive when a subject is sitting or standing, apparently because of good balancing of the skull on the column. The longus is a strong flexor, acting reciprocally with the longissimus, a strong extensor (Fountain et al., 1966). Their influence on lateral bending appears to be minimal, contrary to widespread belief.

The slightest attempt of a supine subject to raise his head recruits marked activity in the sternomastoid and scalenes. We have already noted their respiratory function in Chapter 10.

Mandibular Movements

When the mouth is opened, a hinge-like movement occurs between the head of the mandible and the fibrocartilaginous disc that divides the jaw joint into an upper and a lower compartment (fig. 15.3). At the same time a gliding movement occurs whereby both disc and head move forward (and somewhat downward) on the convex articular eminence of the temporal bone. The lateral pterygoid muscle is attached partly to the anterior capsule (and thus to the disc) and

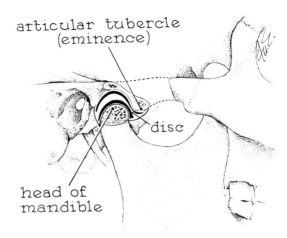

a. Mouth closed

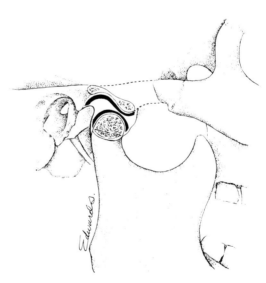

b. Mouth open

Fig. 15.3. Movements of the mandible and its articular disc during simple closing and opening of the mouth.

partly to the neck of the mandible; undoubtedly it provides a major force for the forward glide.

The jaw can also be moved from side to side (as in chewing), a movement involving a shuttling of the two mandibular heads with their discs in the concave parts of the sockets. This shuttling becomes progressively less as the mouth is opened. Grinding actions (circular) involve movements in both axes and in both compartments of the jaw joint.

Forward dislocation is prevented by a limiting ligament, the temporomandibular, the fibres of which are gradually tensed as the mouth is opened. It is simply a thickening of the lateral part of the joint capsule (see also TEMPORALIS, below).

Muscles

Muscles are not the only motive force in mandibular movements; weight (gravity) acts to depress the front of the mandible so that the lower incisors can move forward below the upper incisors, as the reader can verify easily. In opening/closing of the mouth and protraction/retraction of the mandible any three of six forces can come into play. These are the weight of the mandible (W) and five pairs of muscles: the external (lateral) pterygoids (E), the digastrics (D), the masseters (M), the internal (medial) pterygoids (I) and the temporal muscles (T). Their initial letters form the mnemonic word WEDMIT and they cooperate as shown in the scheme in fig. 15.4.

The forceful movements of the jaw are produced by cooperative activity of several muscles bilaterally or unilaterally. Mandibular elevation is performed by the temporalis, masseter and medial pterygoids, and depression by the lateral pterygoids and digastrics. The digastrics show their greatest activity in forceful opening of the mouth at the limit of depression of the mandible. Lateral movements are performed by the ipsilateral temporalis and masseter and the contralateral medial pterygoid (and, to a lesser extent, the lateral

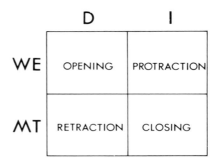

Fig. 15.4. Scheme of mandibular movements and muscles.

pterygoid). Protraction is performed by the medial and lateral pterygoids while retraction is by the temporalis, chiefly its posterior fibres, and perhaps the deep part of masseter.

CO-ORDINATION DURING CHEWING. Variation of pattern is the rule (Ahlgren, 1966). The most common pattern during gum-chewing is one in which the ipsilateral temporalis contracts first, then the contralateral temporalis and both masseters simultaneously. The peak of activity and the ending of activity occur simultaneously most of the time. With peanut-chewing, the most common pattern is that both masseters and temporalis contract simultaneously.

TEMPORALIS. Both the anterior and posterior fibres of temporalis are continuously active in the upright posture. Indeed this muscle is the main postural muscle. For end-to-end (incisor) bite all parts of temporalis are active (contrary to the view of some earlier writers). During molar occlusion all parts of temporalis are markedly active, this being a chief function of the muscle. The posterior fibres retract the jaw but no part of the muscle aids in protraction. Each temporalis pulls the mandible to its own side, acting reciprocally with its homologue during side-to-side movements. During maximal opening of the mouth, the temporalis acts to prevent dislocation along with the temporomandibular ligament.

MASSETER. During forced centric occlusion this muscle is predictably very active. During chewing movements, its maximal activity occurs at about the time the jaw reaches the temporary position of centric occlusion. Not important as a postural muscle, it does show some activity when weight is attached to the mandible (Carlsöö, 1952). It also acts as an ipsilateral abductor of the mandible and helps in its protraction (superficial fibres) and retraction (deep fibres).

MEDIAL PTERYGOID. During simple protraction there is always strong activity in this muscle (Moyers, 1950); this decreases if the mandible is simultaneously depressed. Unilateral activity draws the mandible to the opposite side; the activity is greater if protraction is added.

LATERAL PTERYGOID. During mandibular depression, the first activity appears in the lateral pterygoid and reaches its peak even before the other muscles become active. It continues throughout the whole movement (Moyers, 1950). It is also an important contralateral abductor of the mandible, and a protractor (Woelfel et al., 1960).

DIGASTRIC. During mandibular depression the digastric muscle comes into action rather late, but at this time its action appears to be essential for the maximum depression of forced or complete opening of the mouth and for assisting the lateral pterygoid in moving the chin along the properly curved path. The muscle always seems to act with its partner of the opposite side, never as an individual. Digastric also plays an important rôle in retrusion of the mandible.

Movements of Tongue and Hyoid Bone

The bulk of the tongue is muscular but not all of the muscle fibres are attached to bone. The intrinsic muscles are arranged in three planes—longitudinal, transverse and vertical. By sometimes delicate and sometimes coarse contractions in different combinations they continually alter the shape of this changeable organ. Four extrinsic muscles (styloglossus, hyoglossus, genioglossus and palatoglossus) pull the tongue in different directions. These are all well-known movements and the general function of the various muscles is quite obvious.

What is not known with any degree of accuracy is the precise rôle of the muscles during many specific functions. Indeed the little electromyography that has been reported has cast doubt on well accepted functions. For example, protrusion of the tongue does not recruit genioglossus muscle except when the tongue is pushed against the back of the incisor teeth (Bole, 1965).

During *swallowing* a complex pattern of activity appears in geniohyoid and genioglossus. The movements both of the tongue and of the hyoid bone are not the simple set one finds in textbooks. Thus, during the swallowing of saliva or of water, a pattern of activity has been found which varies between subjects and even between successive swallows by the same subject. Nevertheless, a general pattern is recognizable with clear differences between the swallowing of saliva and the swallowing of water. Even during the brief span of a swallow, the muscles show rapid variations in their contributions from moment to moment (Cunningham and Basmajian, 1968; Hrycyshyn and Basmajian, 1972).

Movements of the Eyeball

These muscles and some of their coordinated functions were discussed briefly in Chapter 6. Fig. 15.5 summarizes the general actions of the various groups. Here we shall add only such information as has been derived from direct experiments.

NORMAL POSITION. The eyeball is maintained in its normal position during waking hours (even in total darkness) by the continuous activity of the recti. Each change in ocular fixation is accompanied by an increase of activity in a prime mover with reciprocal decrease or inhibition of antagonist(s). This occurs whether the movement is slow or fast. With extreme positions of gaze, *e.g.* far to one side or another, the antagonist is usually completely inhibited.

During very fast movements, the prime mover gives one or more sharp bursts of activity while the antagonists are completely inhibited.

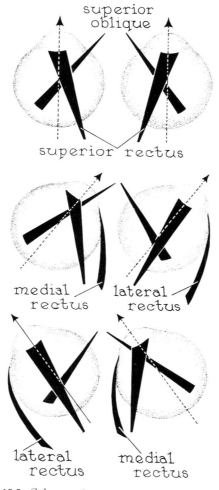

Fig. 15.5. Scheme of eye movements and muscles.

OCULAR REST POSITION. During sleep and surgical anesthesia a convergent depressed position of the eyeball is common. Electromyographic evidence, indicates that the extra-ocular muscles all completely relax in these states.

REFERENCES

Ahlgren, J. (1966). Mechanism of mastication: a quantitative cinematographic and electromyographic study of masticatory movements in children, with special reference to occlusion of the teeth. *Acta Odont. Scandinav.. 24:* suppl. 44, 109 pp.

Bole, C.R. (1965). Electromyographic kinesiology of the genioglossus muscles in man. M.S. Thesis, Ohio State University, Columbus, Ohio.

Carlsöö, S. (1952). Nervous coordination and mechanical function of the mandibular elevators: an electromyographic study of the activity and an anatomic analysis of the mechanics of the muscles. *Acta Odont. Scandinav.. 10:* suppl. 11, 1-132.

Cunningham, D.P. and Basmajian, J.V. (1968). Electromyography of tongue muscles. *Proc. Can. Fed. Biol. Soc.. 11:* 15.

Fountain, F.P., Minear, W.L. and Allison, R.D. (1966). Function of longus colli and longissimus cervicis muscles in man. *Arch. Phys. Med.. 47:* 665-669.

Hrycyshyn, A.W. and Basmajian, J.V. (1972). Electromyography of the oral stage of swallowing in man. Am. J. Anat., 133: 333-340.

Møller, E. (1966). *The Chewing Apparatus.* Copenhagen.

Moyers, R.E. (1950). An electromyographic analysis of certain muscles involved in temporomandibular movement. *Am. J. Orthodontics. 36:* 481-515.

Woelfel, J.B., Hickey, J.C., Stacy, R.W. and Rinear, L. (1960). Electromyographic analysis of jaw movements. *J. Prosthet. Dent.. 10:* 688-697.

SIXTEEN

Applications and Problems

The applications of kinesiology can be divided into industrial and medical, having to do with the healthy and the sick, respectively. The industrial applications fall within the sphere of ergonomics, the adaptation of machines, space and processes to those who work with their hands and/or their feet. In older days men, women and even children were expected to adapt themselves to the machines they served and to the space, however cramped, they were given to toil in. Factory was the tyrant over folk, and the souls and bodies of the common people were crushed and killed by it. No man has epitomized the thing better than Thomas Hood in his *Song of the Shirt*.

Then came Jules Amar, the pioneer in the inquiry into how effort and achievement are related. His work led to those time-and-motion studies that are so widespread today and that still form the basis of attempted reform of work-processes and working conditions. The intention is praiseworthy, the effect less so, for the introduction of new "drills" at the workbench or on the factory floor has too often led to increased rather than decreased fatigue of the workmen or workwomen. This is not surprising.

Ergonomic Cycles

Modern industrial work, particularly of the conveyer-belt type, is largely repetitive. In other words, it can be analysed

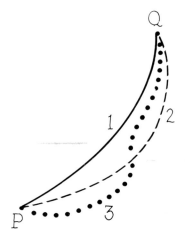

Fig. 16.1. Pathways between an initial point P and an end point Q of a line of motion of a bone. 1, Shortest path (chord); 2, simple arc; 3, sinuous arc.

into a set of repeated work-cycles or *ergonomic cycles*. In general, each cycle consists of three stages, which we may call the *preparatory*, the *operative* and the *return* stages. Suppose the task is the insertion of a screw into some object. First the screw must be obtained from some store, say a box, and brought to the object—preparatory stage. Next it must be inserted in and screwed into the object—operative stage. Lastly the hand must be returned to the store to pick up another screw—return stage. Leaving aside any consideration of the operative stage, it is clear that both the preparatory and the return stages call for movements at the shoulder, elbow, forearm and wrist joints. At none of these joints does any bone move through space in a straight line (Chapter 4), nor will they usually move in the shortest possible (chordal) line from starting point to end point (Chapter 4), but in arcuate lines. There is, in fact, an infinity of possible arcuate lines when the joints have 2 or 3 degrees of freedom, as at the wrist and shoulder, respectively. Every man will have some particular lines of motion which he finds most comfortable for the

performance of some part of a repeated task. These lines may
be simple arcs or sinuous arcs (fig. 16.1), but whichever they
are he should not be asked to change them without careful
consideration of other aspects of ergonomic cycles that we
shall now go into.

The paramount fact about an ergonomic cycle is that every
bone involved in it moves in a closed diadochal path (Chapter
4). This has three "legs". The first leg is that of the preparatory stage, the second is that of the operative stage and the
third is that of the return stage. These three legs form a trigone (Chapter 4). Furthermore, at the end of the cycle every
bone is again in the posture it was in at the beginning of the
cycle, for this is what a "cycle" means. Hence the sum of the
three internal angles of the trigone must be 180° (Chapter 4).
Lastly, the shape of the legs of the trigone is of no consequence provided that the condition just mentioned is fulfilled.
This is illustrated in fig. 16.2, a and b. In a each leg of the
cycle is simple, whereas in b the operative leg is quite complex as would be the case in some complicated task carried
out by the working hand. But in each case the sum of the
angles A, B and C is the same—two right angles, and the first
and last states of the bone involved are the same in each case.

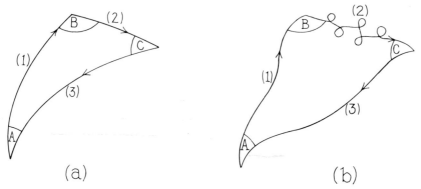

Fig. 16.2. Two types of ergonomic cycle. In each case (1) is the preparatory stage, (2) the operative stage and (3) the return stage, and the sum of
the angles A, B and C is 180°. Further details are given in the text.

Of course, the worker knows nothing about the angles A, B and C, nor does he give any conscious attention to the shape of the first and third stages of the ergonomic cycles of the bones he moves. But we know that *he has 2 degrees of freedom in carrying out the movements of his hand*, for this is a consequence of the fact that (A + B + C) = 180°. Assuming that his movements during the operative stage of the cycle are determined by the nature of his work and are, as it were, dictated to him, then he is free to shape the first and last legs of the ergonomic cycle as he pleases. He is like a Canadian who has to make some prescribed journey within Mexico but is free both to reach and to return from that country by any route that he pleases. Indeed, this simile pinpoints the two aspects which require consideration in any time-and-motion study of any ergonomic cycle: (1) that the cycle should be considered *as a whole* in any given instance, and (2) that the motion should be studied before the time taken to accomplish it.

The kinematic rule governing any ergonomic cycle is simply this: *The sum of all the conjunct rotations within the cycle is zero.* This is the succinct way of expressing in words what is contained in the equation (A + B + C) = 180°. Some of these conjunct rotations arise from the fact that the habitual motions at our joints are usually arcuate, not chordal. Others are consequential, arising from the fact that the movements of the "working" limb are in fact diadochal movements, as these have been defined in Chapter 4. These diadochal movements may not be adverted to, may even be unsuspected; but they do occur and must be undone sooner or later. Consequently, what might seem an unduly complex motion in the return stage of a cycle is really one that is essential for undoing the effects of one or more conjunct rotations that have occurred in the two preceding stages. In particular, should the worker's choice of movement(s) in the preparatory stage cause any conjunct rotation(s) not undone in the operative stage, then the return stage of motion will have to depart from what some observers might recommend as being simpler at first sight.

Although we are inexpert in ergonomics we venture to suggest certain applications of what has been said so far.

There is a place for studies of what acceptedly good workmen actually do when performing specific tasks that are repeated again and again. The object of these studies would not be to look for "remediable faults" but to discover the range of variation that should be allowed for in the conclusions to be drawn in any further motion studies. A skilled worker is one who performs his tasks without unnecessary fatigue of his muscles, but he and he alone is competent to judge how he is to do it. As we have shown in our chapters on special kinesiology, there is often considerable difference between individuals with respect to the muscles actually used in such a simple operation as flexion of the elbow, notwithstanding the fact that all were tested under precisely similar conditions. How much the more, then, may we expect differences in the use of the musculature of a whole limb when the hand is being brought to or away from its locus of operation. These differences in muscular usage may well show themselves in differences in the preparatory and return paths of motion. It is not suggested that even a good workman may not be trained to use his muscles better. But those who make the suggestions should do so by example as well as by precept, and the example should be based on a testing period of performance of the "better" way over a span of time commensurate with that for which the workman has to work.

Our second application follows from the first. One should always remember that the bones, joints and muscles of the upper limb (for example) are only the servants of the hand. It is the hand that does the actual work; the other parts are merely modes of conveying the hand from place to place or, in many cases, of supplying it with the energy that is involved, say, in hammering a nail. With the hand we should include the radius, for the upper limb consists of two overlapping major parts: the humero-ulnar and the radio-manual. These two parts articulate "in parallel" at the radio-ulnar joints*.

But the trunk is usually involved as well, supplementing the actions of the shoulder girdle, and the lower limbs also in a standing man. Thus rotations in the vertebral column and hip can, and often do, play their part in determining the actual pathway of a working hand. Up to a point there is total involvement of the body in every normal action of the natural man, a sharing of effort between a multitude of muscles and of joints. It can be as tiring and as painful to be constrained to stillness as to be constrained to continual gymnastics—as our modern torturers know! Hence the importance of ensuring that a man's working space shall be sufficient to allow him room to move himself as well as his hands.

In this connection we would mention the importance of modern physical anthropology. We all know about tall folk and short folk, long heads and round heads, and that millions have been murdered because their noses had the "wrong" shape. But it is even more important to realize that limbs and segments of limbs can vary considerably from one group of people to another, both in absolute and in relative length. This has a direct bearing upon the "reach of the hand" from person to person, therefore upon the amount by which the body must supplement the motions of the arm during the various stages of an ergonomic cycle. We make the point and leave it.

Turning now to the time aspect of time-and-motion studies, we would repeat that this should come second and not first. The time taken for the *whole* work-cycle matters more (we think) than the time taken for any one part of it in isolation. Here we are up against the question of "personal rhythms" and the complementary question of work-breaks. Every man has his private *optimal* timing of action, that which enables

---

* The lower limb, on the contrary, consists of two major parts that articulate "in series": the femoral and the cruropedal, joined at the knee.

him to dig or hammer or cut to the best effect over a period of work. We would stress the word "optimal" which is not by any means always the same as *adagio* or *prestissimo!* It would seem that the optimal range for most folk is between *andante* and *allegro*. These differences in personal rhythm would seem to arise from differences in the working of the central nervous system, to which all our muscles are in slavery, for they themselves contract when ordered to. But whatever their cause, these differences exist.

This has a bearing upon many aspects of industrial conditions, especially in those trades concerned in feverish export drives in which a continuously high level of production is called for. Here the workers form an orchestra whose conductor is the conveyer-belt or its equivalent. Now those in an orchestra must not only keep in tune but they must also keep in time. The more a player is at heart an artist the more will he find it difficult to keep in strict time with his fellows, for the score is the text but the pace is the interpretation of the text. To keep an imposed time, then, may be tiring. The great composers of the late 18th and early 19th centuries seem to have sensed this. In their concerti they provided rest periods for both the virtuoso and the others in the form of the *cadenza*, during which the virtuoso could play what he pleased within the general framework of the themes while the others kept silent: he had relative rest; the others had absolute rest.

It is even so for men in general. During a working day they need times of both absolute and relative rest. It is with the latter that we are concerned in this book. To use the current jargon, a man is not hardware but software. Sleep may knit up the ravelled sleeve of care, yet not by sleep alone do men recuperate but by exercise as well: recreation is indeed recreation. Harvey, as great and as immortal a genius as Newton, founded physiology when he wrote upon the motions of the heart and of the blood. Today we know that these depend in no small way upon the motions of our muscles and our joints. The venous pumps of the limbs and body wall are essential for maintaining a good circulation and for the health of the whole man: haemorrhoids may be caused by livers or by laziness! These venous pumps are worked by the pressures of muscles swelling as they contract: it is they that squeeze the blood from one intervalvular segment of a vein into another.

If, then, a man be restricted in the motions he makes in the course of his work he will be the worse for it sooner or later unless he compensates in some way. This way could take the form of playing some vigorous game in his free time; watching a ball-game or driving an automobile is no substitute. Or it could take the form of some different kind of work, alternating with the other during his working hours. Longfellow's village blacksmith led a more healthy life than his urban successors of our day. We allow the poet the last word.

Medical Applications

The detailed study of muscles and motions, as we have tried to present it, has so many obvious medical applications that we shall not insult the reader by listing them in full. Yet it is useful to classify them as threefold: diagnostic, therapeutic and educative, and the last is really first. We can think without muscles, notwithstanding the Behaviourist dogma: ask anyone who has been medically curarized. But our whole action upon the world is by means of them and they have a corresponding claim on our attention. As lately (or remotely?) as our own student days the forms, origins and insertions of muscles were a bugbear to the learner, largely meaningless and of no great clinical significance. The same was true of the detailed structure of the joints. The advance, first of orthopaedics then of physical medicine, has changed all that. Even if a student does not intend to become a specialist in either of these fields he should be given some notion of what is possible in the way of diagnosis and therapy and even learn to practise some parts of these by himself. Apart from medical men, however, there are the physiotherapists whose whole work is founded upon musculature and movement. In Ireland

and Britain, anyway, these are not allowed to work except under medical direction—are the blind to lead those who can see?*

We have now both a growing experimental knowledge of the locomotor system and an expanding theory for ordering it understandably. We are better fitted now to discriminate between what all students should know and what more only some must know. Empirical learning can now be replaced by scientific, as has already happened in the case of all other systems of the body. The theory may well be modified as facts accumulate; meanwhile it could serve as a basis for directed rather than haphazard research, for stimulating rather than soporific teaching.

The remedial side has been well dealt with by the contributors to Sidney Licht's *Therapeutic Exercise* (1961), now available in several languages. Here, as in the realm of diagnosis, there is a large overlap of orthopaedic surgery and physical medicine and room for abundant, fertile coöperation. Diagnosis and aetiology are so closely (though not wholly) linked that what every advance in the second of these adds is a greater surety to the first. This brings us to our final matter, that of problems.

Problems

On the medical as on the industrial side one problem to be solved is that of the normal range of variation in the use of particular muscles for bringing about given movements— elbow flexion, hip abduction and so on. The principles of minimal action (Chapter 7) are hypotheses backed by a considerable amount of experimental evidence, but their general applicability still remains to be tested. It is important that it should be tested, for once the extent of its domain is known we shall have a means of distinguishing those who use

---

* Sometimes they can. It was a blind man who guided the customers of a department store to the street (in Hamilton, Ontario) during the famous blackout of 1965!

muscles normally and those who do not. This in turn will help in the diagnosis of neuromuscular disorders.

The next problem is that of finding out whether the musculature that brings about some motion at a single joint in isolation is the same as that which brings about the same motion when other joints in series with it are also moved. We have recorded above some work of this kind in connection with the fingers and the feet, but there is very much more to be done. Cognate with this problem is that of the influence of the position in space of a *stabilized* joint upon the selection and strength of the muscles used to keep it stable. Suppose, for example, that a forearm is first flexed to 45° upon a pendent humerus and is then kept stabilized while the humerus is flexed to some new position. This causes the forearm to assume a new position relative to the line of action of gravity. Does the musculature acting on the elbow change or remain the same? The theory propounded in Chapter 7 suggests that a change takes place in at least the total strength of the operative musculature—but the theory may be wrong!

Yet another field of future research lies simply in testing the truth of results already published by others. In these days of *Publish or perish!* the search for newness imperils the search for trueness. We would stress the fact that kinesiology is today at about the same stage as was chemistry well over a hundred years ago. The triumphs of modern chemistry stem as much from assiduous exercises of verification as from the brilliant flashes of inspiration of the Kekulés and the Mendeleëvs. We shall have to take this lesson to heart and remember that attempts at verification (or disproof) apply as much to experimental data as to hypotheses designed to explain these data. There is ample work to be done in this field alone.

Cognate with the problem of verification is that of the correlation of intramuscular electromyography with the "surface-electrode" type. Inserted fine-wire EMG is undoubtedly the only form that will give *full* information about how muscles actually work: both original and verificatory work must be based upon it. But it does involve both a piercing of the skin and a very detailed knowledge of anatomy. Both these considerations restrict its use in general clinical practice, including physiotherapy. Hence the need to discover whether *adequate* (as distinct from full) information can be obtained by the simpler method. In other words, the problem is whether we can provide a "dictionary" by means of which the results obtained from "epidermic" EMG can be translated into those of "hypodermic" EMG.

Finally there is the problem of the unapproachable muscles, those that cannot be reached either because of their situation or because of the dangers attendant upon experiment. The subscapularis is an example of the latter kind. It can be reached by needle-electrodes but, it has been found, the venous plexuses of the axilla are easily injured, giving rise to haematomas. This is impermissible when we are dealing with human beings, volunteers or not. To such muscles we must apply reasoning from a knowledge of their origins and insertions and of well-attested theory. Every branch of knowledge has its fringe of the directly inaccessible. Kinesiology is no exception.

REFERENCE

Licht, S. (1961). *Therapeutic Exercise*. Elizabeth Licht, New Haven, Conn.

The Geometry and Algebra of Articular Kinematics

By M. A. MacConaill

THE GEOMETRY OF SURFACES

The kinematics of bones and joints can be reduced to motions on some surface or other. Hence we begin with an account of the relevant geometry of surfaces.

1.1. We distinguish three types of surface: the *ovoid*, the *flat* and the *sellar*.

An ovoid surface is one that is either wholly concave or wholly convex. A sellar surface is one that is convex in one direction and becomes concave as the direction (plane of section) rotates through a right angle; the articular surfaces of a saddle-joint are like this, hence the name "sellar". A flat surface is one that is either a plane or formed by rolling a plane surface up to form a cone or cylinder.*

1.2. The shortest line (or path) between any two points on a surface will be called a *chord*. Any other line wholly on the surface between the chosen points, whatever be its shape, will be called an *arc*.

---

* The terms ovoid and sellar were introduced (MacConaill, 1946) as easily understood substitutes for "synclastic" and "anticlastic", respectively. A flat surface can also be called "aclastic".

(Reprinted from *Bio-Medical Engineering* (April, 1966), London, England, by kind permission of the Editorial Board.)

1.2.1. The facts of arthrology entitle us to assume that there is only one chord between any two points on the surfaces we have to consider. This chord corresponds to a straight line on a plane. The term chord is familiar as a correlative to arc; it is preferable to "geodesic", which term is also applied to the longest distance between two points.

1.3. A *triangle* is a closed, three-sided figure, all the sides of which are chords.

The *residual* (r) of a triangle is defined thus: Let s be the sum of the three interior angles of a triangle; then

$$r = s - \pi$$

For any ovoid surface s is greater than π, so that r is positive; for a flat surface s is equal to π, so that r is zero; for a sellar surface s is less than π, so that r is negative. Hence ovoid, flat and sellar surfaces are also called surfaces of positive, zero (or null) and negative curvature, respectively.

Instances of the three types of surface and of the corresponding types of triangle are shown in fig. A.1.

1.3.1. On an ovoid or sellar surface—but not on a flat—the absolute (*i.e.* arithmetical) value of the residual increases

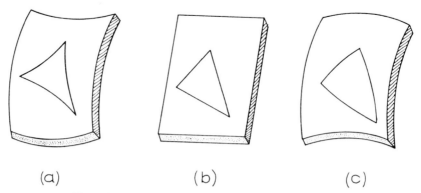

(a)   (b)   (c)

Fig. A.1. Triangles on sellar, flat and ovoid surfaces (a, b and c respectively).

with the area of the triangle, and conversely. This can be proved by a set of simple exercises in finite geometry.

Take, for example, the triangle (1, 2, 3) on an ovoid surface shown in fig. A.2. This triangle is divided into two others, (1, 2, 2') and (1, 2', 3). The triangle (1, 2, 3) has a sum (s) of interior angles that is ($a + d + c + e$). The corresponding sum (s') for the smaller triangle (1, 2', 3) is ($a + b + c$). The triangle (1, 2, 2') has a sum of angles ($d + e + f$). Now in all geometries the sum of the two adjacent angles where one line cuts another is always π. Hence ($b + f$) = π, so that ($b + f$) is less than ($d + e + f$). We have thus:

$d + e > b$ whence ($a + d + e + c$) > ($a + b + c$)

whence $s > s'$ and ($s - \pi$) > ($s' - \pi$)

That is, $r > r'$ so that r' is nearer to 0 than r. The reader should verify that r' is nearer to 0 than r in the corresponding case when the surface is a sellar one, remembering that r is less than ($b + f$).

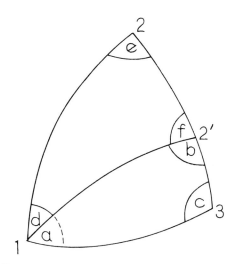

Fig. A.2. To illustrate section (1.3.1) in text.

1.4 An n-sided closed figure, all the sides of which are chords, can be called a *multangle*—by analogy with a triangle. Such a figure can be divided into $(n - 2)$ triangles having a common apex, from which it can be shown easily that the residual of a multangle is given by: $r = s - (n - 2)\pi$, in which equation s is the sum of the interior angles of the multangle. The reader should verify this for a 4-sided and a 5-sided figure. These two cases and that of the triangle are sufficient to establish the rule by mathematical induction.

1.5. A *trigone* is a closed, 3-sided figure having at least one side that is not a chord. Similarly a *polygone* is a closed, n-sided figure having at least one side that is not a chord.

The residual of an n-sided figure is defined exactly as is that of multangle. But, unlike the figures formed by chords, the sum of the interior angles of the n-gone may be equal to, greater than or less than $(n - 2)\pi$, whatever be the type of surface on which it lies.

When this sum is precisely $(n - 2)\pi$ then the figure is called *Euclidean*, for it has the residual (*i.e.* 0) of any n-sided multangle in Euclidean geometry.

1.6. If an arc and a chord (or two arcs) join the same two points on a surface then we have a *digone* in which $n = 2$. It follows from (1.4) that the residual of a digone is equal to the algebraic sum of the two internal angles of the digone.

1.7. *The residual of a chord is zero.* This theorem is both meaningful and true because any chord is the limiting case of a set of triangles having that chord as their common base.

Referring again to fig. A.2, if the chord $(1, 3)$ be the chord in question then as the chord $(1, 2')$ is drawn nearer and nearer to the chord $(1, 3)$ so does r' become nearer and nearer to 0, taking this value in the limit when $2'$ and 3 do coincide.

This property is a necessary but not sufficient datum for the proof that the curvature of a chord is null, a theorem to be proved later.

TYPES OF MOVEMENT ON SURFACES

2.1. Movements on surfaces are studied by means of a *rodlet*. This is an infinitesimal rod on which, however, three distinct points can be distinguished: a head, a middle and a tail. The rod is assumed to be tangent to the surface, the tangency taking place at the middle of the rod (fig. A.3, *ii*). A rodlet can be represented by an arrow, the "barb" of which is at the head of the rodlet.

2.2. A rodlet can perform either or both of two kinds of motion on the surface: *spin* and *slide*.

2.3. Spin is a partial or complete rotation of the rodlet about a normal (perpendicular) to the surface that passes through the midpoint of the rodlet.
    "Spin" is used instead of the more ambiguous term "rotation" of ordinary mechanics.

2.3.1. A spin of angle a is signified by E^a. This angle may be positive, negative or zero. If a clockwise spin be called positive then an anticlockwise spin is negative.
    The symbol E^a corresponds to the symbol e^{ia} of complex-variable algebra.

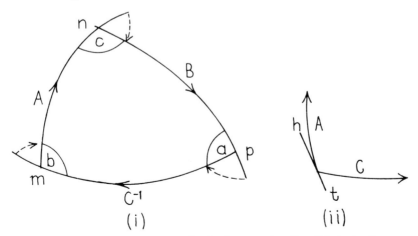

Fig. A.3. To illustrate the basic theorem (section 3.1 in text).

2.3.2. $A^a \cdot E^b = E^{a \cdot b}$

2.3.3. $E^0 = I$

The sign $=$ signifies "is equivalent to" and the sign I signifies "no motion".

2.3.4. $E^{2n\pi} = E^0 = I$.

This is because a spin through a full circle (2π) restores the rodlet to its original orientation and is, therefore, equivalent to no motion at all.

Example: $E^{3\pi} = E^{2\pi} \cdot E^{\pi} = IE^{\pi} = E^{\pi}$.

2.3.5.   If a spin E^a takes place at a point m on the surface we write $m E^a m$ to indicate this fact.

2.4.   Slide is any motion of the rodlet along some pathway on the surface, the sliding point being the midpoint of the rodlet.

The term "slide" is used instead of "translation" to indicate that the motion is wholly upon the surface in question.

2.4.1. A slide from a point m along a path A to a point n is signified by mAn.

2.4.2. Two successive slides, mAn and nBp, are signified thus:

$$mAn \cdot nBp = mABp$$

2.4.3. Such algebraic forms as mAn and nBp are called *triads*. Every such triad represents a finite vector, *i.e.* a finite line that has a direction, *e.g.* from m to n. The triad $mE^a m$ represents a spin-vector.

The equation (2.4.2) is an instance of the composition of triads. The form AB corresponds to the $(A + B)$ of ordinary mechanics but is a more useful one in our present kinematics. No metrical implications are contained in the form AB. It is a geometrical form, *i.e.* belonging to that branch of mathematics that takes no account of non-angular metrical concepts other than "equal to", "greater than" and "less than", as in Euclid's Elements. The symbol AB is to be read "A followed by B".

No two triads can be composed unless the last member of

the first is identical with the first member of the second. This restriction expresses the fact that the rodlet cannot leave the surface and "jump" from one point to another.

2.4.4. If we have mAn then the precisely reverse slide is shown by $nA^{-1}m$.

2.4.5. $mAn \cdot nA^{-1}m = mAA^{-1}m = mA^0m = mIm$.

That is to say, A and A^{-1} are inverses to each other and their composition is equivalent to no motion at all.

2.5. $mAn \cdot nE^a n = mAE^a n = mE^a m \cdot mAn = mE^a An$

That is, a spin and a slide can be combined, and the order of composition is immaterial to the result. The spin could, of course, take place during the slide, but the end result would be the same as if each took place separately.

2.5.1. $mE^a m \cdot mAn \cdot nBp \cdot pE^b p = mE^{a+b}ABp = mABE^{a+b}p$.

This theorem is a consequence of (2.5). It shows that we can bring all spin vectors together (regardless of their order) and all slide vectors together (provided their order be strictly preserved). In other words, spin vectors commute with all vectors but slide vectors commute only with spin vectors.

2.5.2. Let mAp be a given slide and let n be a point on A between m and p. Then we have:

$$mAp = mAn \cdot nAp \quad \text{and hence}$$
$$mAp \cdot pA^{-1}n = mAn.$$

This example shows that we cannot reduce the left-hand side of the second equation to mIn. This accords with common sense, for m and n are different points. The first equation shows that $mA^2p = mAp$ provided that the composition of the two triads involved is permissible by (2.4.3.). The two equations indicate that the algebra of our kinematics is one form of Boolean algebra.

2.6. Let $mABC^{-1}E^r m = mIm$.

Then $AB = CE^{-r}$ by transposition of terms and $mABn = mCE^{-r}n$.

That is to say, the *equipollent* (or true equivalent) of the two-stage slide from m to n is not the one-stage slide C between the same points but that one-stage slide together with the spin E^{-r}.

This shows that it is possible for two slides to be equivalent to a single slide together with a spin. The importance of this theorem for articular kinematics will be shown in (3.1).

2.6.1. In elementary kinematics one considers the movement of a *point* (or particle). Spin is not taken into account. Hence if we had $mABn$ and mCn we should write $AB = C$; that is, C would be considered the kinematic, though not necessarily the kinetic, equivalent of AB. The reader will recall that kinematics treats of motions alone, whereas kinetics takes account also of the forces and energies associated with motions. But spin must be taken into account in the kinematics of a rodlet, as will be shown in (3.1).

2.6.2. In the movements of points or particles upon a surface only the displacement of the points or particles is in question; hence, if we have both $mABp$ and mCp we are justified in calling C the resultant of AB. In the movements of rodlets, however, we are also concerned with the orientation of the rodlets as a result of the displacements. Hence, in general, not C but CE^r would represent the effect of AB. We shall therefore distinguish between resultants and equipollents, the former term referring to displacements alone, the latter referring to displacement and orientation combined.

Anticipating what is to be said about the actual movements of bones and at joints, we shall refer to the combination of locus and orientation of a rodlet as its *posture.*

Finally, it will be shown that there is an important class of instances in which resultants are also equipollents.

2.7. Two or more successive slides will be called a *diadochal movement,* from the Greek *diadochos* (successive).

Thus AB, ABC $(ABC\ldots N)$ represent diadochal movements.

2.8. A single slide will be called a *monodal* movement, from *monos* (single) and *hodos* (path).

2.9. The definitions and theorems of this section complete the necessary and sufficient algebra for all that follows.

THE GENERAL KINEMATICS OF SURFACES

The general kinematics of surfaces is derived from a basic theorem:

3.1. Let a closed trigone of sliding motion have the sides mAn, nBp and $pC^{-1}m$, as shown in fig. A.3; let the internal angles opposite A, B and C be a, b and c, respectively; and let r be the residual of the trigone: then $AB = CE^r$.

That is: A diadochal movement between two points on any surface is equivalent to a monodal path between the same two points together with a spin, the magnitude and sense of which are that of the residual of the trigone formed by the diadochal and monodal paths combined.

Proof: Place a rodlet at m so that it points along A, as shown in fig. 125, *ii*. Slide it to n in such a way that it always points along (is tangent to) A. At n, spin it through the angle $(\pi - c)$; it will now point along B. Slide it along B to p and then make it point along C^{-1} by making it spin through an angle $(\pi - a)$. Finally, slide it along C^{-1} to m and spin it through an angle $(\pi - b)$; it will now be in its original posture on the surface. We have, therefore:

$$mAE^{\pi-c}n \cdot nBE^{\pi-a}p \cdot pC^{-1}E^{\pi-b}m = mIm$$

Putting s for $(a + b + c)$ and remembering that $E^{3\pi} = E^{\pi}$, we find:

$$ABC^{-1}E^{3\pi-s} = ABC^{-1}E^{\pi-s} = ABC^{-1}E^{-r} = I$$

$$AB = CE^r$$

which proves the theorem.

3.2. The spin E^r in the basic theorem is called a *conjunct spin* because it is necessarily conjoined with the diadochal movement AB.

3.3. If ABC^{-1} is a clockwise path and r is positive then the conjunct spin is also clockwise. By examining suitable instances we find that the relationship between the sense of the diadochal path, the sense of r and the sense of the rotation is as set out in Table I.

As the table shows, the rule is: *the sense of a conjunct spin is equal to the product of the sense of the diadochal path and the sign of r.*

For example, a clockwise path AB with $r = -20°$ produces an anti-clockwise conjunct spin of magnitude $20°$. An anti-clockwise path AB with $r = -20°$ gives a clockwise conjunct spin of $20°$.

3.2.2. If the trigone is Euclidean, *i.e.* if $r = 0$, then $AB = C$. Hence the resultant of AB is also its equipollent and $ABC^{-1} = I$. This is the theory of ergonomic cycles (MacConaill, 1965), so called because motion of a bone fulfilling this condition completes a work-cycle in some repetitive task.

The general theorem for a diadochal path of $(n - I)$ elements is

$$m(ABC \ldots M)p = mNE^r p$$

$$r = s - (n - 2)\pi.$$

This follows from (3.1) by (1.4).

Table I: C and $-$C indicate clockwise and anti-clockwise motion, respectively.

Sense of diadochal path	Sign of r	Sense of conjunct spin
C	+	C
$-$C	+	$-$C
$\pm$C	0	0
C	$-$	$-$C
$-$C	$-$	C

3.4. The basic theorem is perfectly general. Indeed, as the method of proof shows, it does not take specific account of the surface on which the diadochal path and its monodal resultant lie. But when we have to do with chordal paths, in which A, B and C are the shortest distances between their terminal points, then the nature of the surface is relevant. We must, then, consider the essential kinematic difference between any arc and a chord.

3.5. It has been shown (1.7) that the residual of a chord is zero. Since a chord is the limiting case of a triangle (1.7) it follows that motion along a chord is the limiting case of motion along two sides of a triangle. Suppose we have a triangle (ABC) such that we have the slides $mABp$ and mCp. Then as (A, B, C) degenerates into C so does the conjunct spin proper to AB become smaller and then vanish. That is to say, *a chord is always a path of no conjunct spin.*

It follows that a chord on any surface is the geometrical and kinematical equivalent of a straight line on a plane. It is interesting to note that the proof of this depends upon a kinematical, *i.e.* a physical theorem.

3.6. It follows from the above that a completely chordal (holochordal) diadochal path cannot have a chordal monodal path as its equipollent, unless the surface be flat. If $mABP$ be such a path and if mCp be the chordal resultant thereof then the equipollent path mPb will be an *arc*, as shown in fig. A.4. This arc will be convex *inwards* (inside the triangle of chordal paths) if (A, B, C) has a residual greater than zero, and will be convex *outwards* (outside the chordal triangle) if (A, B, C) has a residual less than zero. In all cases the trigone (A, B, P) will have a residual exactly equal to zero.

3.7. As shown in fig. A.5, an arc mAn may either lie wholly on one side of its proper chord mCn or cross this chord. Passage along the arc will give rise to a conjunct spin of a rodlet. The amount and sense of this spin will depend upon the

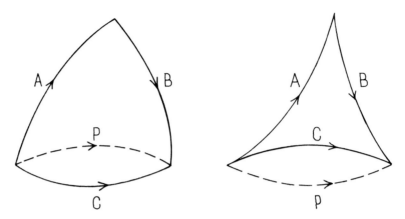

Fig. A.4. To show the equipollents (P) of an ovoid and a sellar diadochal chordal path AB. C is also a chordal path.

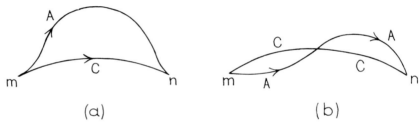

Fig. A.5. Two forms of arc (A) with their proper chords (C).

relation of the arc to the chord, being the algebraic sum of the two angles subtended by the arc with the chord. Depending upon the sign assigned to clockwise rotation (positive or negative), this sum will be either positive or negative if the chord be not crossed by the arc; but if the arc crosses the chord then one angle can be positive and the other negative, thus reducing the magnitude of the conjunct spin. In the latter case the spin may actually be zero, in which case we could call the arc *quasichordal*, for it would be kinematically equivalent to a chord.

3.8. *Curvature of a path.* Following the precedent of plane geometry, we could define the curvature of a path as *the average conjunct spin per unit of length* associated with sliding along it. This entails the consequence that quasichordal arcs could be reckoned to be uncurved! The matter is properly resolved by differential geometry, a procedure quite irrelevant to our purposes. It is for this reason that the terms "chord" and "arc" were chosen for anatomical use.

3.9. *Adjunct spin.* Any spin other than a conjunct spin is called an adjunct spin. In many instances the effect of a conjunct spin can be mitigated, nullified or even changed in sign as well as in magnitude by an adjunct spin.

THE KINEMATICS OF A BONE

All bones move at joints. But the kinematics of a bone does not require any inquiry into the kinematics of the joint at which the bone moves. The bone is considered simply as an object moving in space, an object that can be studied without opening the joint. We are now in the realm of experimental fact.

4.1. There is no loss of generality in considering our bone to be a long bone and in restricting our attention to the shaft of this bone. What is learnt thereby can easily be applied to short and flat bones. Furthermore, we shall confine our study to the motions of a bone in so far as these are dependent upon its movement(s) at a single joint, *e.g.* the radius moving at the elbow.

4.2. The path of any chosen point in or on a bone is always a curved path. The curvature may be slight but it is always present.

4.2.1. The complete set of possible paths of our chosen point constitutes a curved surface. This surface is always convex away from the joint at which the bone moves. It is, therefore, an ovoid surface, and will be called the *ovoid of motion.*

4.3. To study the motion of the bone we select some long axis within the shaft and suppose a rodlet to be attached to this

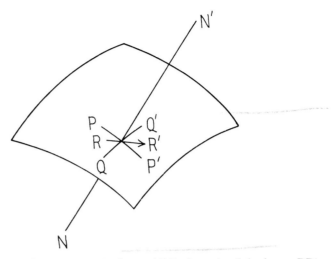

Fig. A.6. An ovoid of motion of a bone. NN′, the axis of the bone. RR′, a rodlet carried on the axis. PP′ and QQ′, two of the paths of motion of the rodlet that generate the ovoid of motion.

axis, making a right angle within it. Thus the actual object of our study is the rodlet as it moves over the ovoid of motion that is generated by the midpoint of the rodlet by its varied movements in space, as is shown in fig. A.6.

Thus the kinematics of the bone is reduced to the kinematics of a rodlet moving on an ovoid surface. Corresponding to each possible movement of the bone there will be a movement of the rodlet, and conversely. The study of *osteokinematics* (as we may call it) consists in working out this one-one correlation in terms applicable to medical problems.

4.4. For all fundamental problems we can imagine the axis of the bone to be indefinitely prolongable. The more the axis is prolonged the more does the ovoid of motion approximate to the surface of a sphere about whose centre the bone-axis rotates in our space. Hence we can use the classical concept of the *sphere of motion* of a bone at a joint for many practical purposes. This cannot be done generally in the case of *intra-articular* kinematics.

4.4.1. Whatever be the shape of the ovoid of motion the bone-axis is always a normal (perpendicular) to it, and the rodlet at the chosen point on the axis is always in a tangent plane to the ovoid of motion.

4.5. *Motions of a bone*. These are of two quite different types: *swings* and *spins*.

4.5.1. Swings of the bone (axis) correspond to slides of the rodlet on the ovoid of motion, and conversely. Swings are either *chordal* or *arcuate*, these terms being derived from the corresponding motions of the rodlet. (But see 4.5.4.)

4.5.2. A spin of the bone, called a *rotation* in medical parlance, corresponds to a spin of the rodlet on the ovoid of motion. A clockwise or anti-clockwise spin will be called a medial or a lateral rotation according to the side on which it occurs and the aspect from which it is viewed. Thus the lateral rotation of a right humerus (shaft) will appear as a clockwise spin to the person carrying out the movement, but as an anti-clockwise spin to one viewing the moving bone from in front.

4.5.3. All movements of a bone are either swings or rotations or combinations of these.

For example, forward flexion and backward extension of the humerus correspond to slides of the rodlet.

Forward flexion and backward extension of the humerus are swings in a vertical plane; abduction and adduction are swings in a vertical plane at right angles to the aforementioned plane; horizontal flexion and horizontal extension are swings in a plane at right angles to both the other two.*

4.5.4. If the bone-shaft moves from its first to its final position by the shortest route it undergoes a *cardinal swing*; this cor-

---

*The terminology used for movements is that adopted by the English-speaking Orthopaedic Associations and published by the American Academy of Orthopaedic Surgeons (1965), later reprinted by the British Orthopaedic Association in 1966. The writer earnestly advocates its general adoption by those who publish matter upon the joints and muscles.

responds to a chordal path of the rodlet on the ovoid of motion. Otherwise the swing is an arcuate swing, corresponding to motion of the rodlet along an arc.

The word "cardinal" is derived from the Latin *cardo* (a hinge).

4.5.5. *Every arcuate swing entails a conjunct spin of the bone.* From now onwards we shall use the word "rotation" instead of "spin" when referring to movements of a bone. Thus we shall refer to conjunct rotations and adjunct rotations as occasion demands.

4.6. We can now define the Degrees of Freedom (DF) of a bone in kinematic terms.

4.6.1. If a bone can swing in two distinct planes and also rotate independently of both these swings then it has 3 DF, for example the humerus.

4.6.2. If a bone can swing in two distinct planes but has no rotation other than conjunct rotation(s) then it has 2 DF. Examples: First metacarpal, first phalanges of fingers.

4.6.3. If a bone can move only in one arcuate swing *or* if it has only adjunct rotation then it has 1 DF.

Examples: Second and third phalanges of fingers, axis vertebra.

No hinge joint permits a cardinal swing; every movement at it involves some conjunct rotation (MacConaill, 1953, 1964).

4.7. At all non-pivot joints the *characteristic* (or habitual) *movement* of a bone is an arcuate swing (MacConaill, 1964, 1965). Thus the humerus and femur tend to rotate laterally when swinging forwards and to rotate medially when swinging backwards.

4.8 If a bone undergoes a cardinal swing in one plane and then a cardinal swing in a different plane it will undergo a *conjunct rotation*. Hence its final posture will be the same as if it had undergone a cardinal swing in a third plane together with a determinable adjunct rotation, or if it had undergone a definable arcuate swing from its first to its final position. This easily verifiable theorem is stated more exactly as follows.

Let mFn, nHp and pAm be three cardinal swings. Compounding them we obtain $mFHAm$; that is, the three cardinal swings will move the bone first away from and finally back to its original position. But they will not bring it back into its original posture. This is because the movements of the corresponding rodlet generate a chordal triangle on the ovoid of motion of the bone. Each side of this chordal triangle is an intersection of a plane of cardinal swing with the ovoid of motion. Thus the internal angles of the triangle are the several *dihedral angles* between the planes taken in pairs. Now the ovoid of motion is, of course, an ovoid surface. Hence the residual of the "triangle of swings" is greater than zero in magnitude. We have then:

$$FHA = E^r \text{ and } FH = A^{-1}E^r$$

This explains the occurrence of the rotation. The sense of the rotation will be that in which the closed path is traversed.

The humerus furnishes an example. If F, H and A stand for forward flexion, horizontal extension and adduction respectively, then the diadochal cardinal swing FH brings the limb (not permitted to move otherwise) into the same posture as it would have had by undergoing abduction (A^{-1}) and lateral rotation. This example is fully discussed and illustrated in Barnett, Davies and MacConaill (1961), in which it is shown that forward flexion through a right angle followed by a horizontal extension of the same amount brings the limb into a position of abduction through a right angle together with lateral rotation through a right angle—these last two values being predictable from the first two.

4.8.1 This phenomenon of conjunct rotation because of diadochal swing (cardinal or otherwise) is of major importance in functional anatomy and its applications. It applies, for example, to movements of the eyeball and serves to explain the presence of the two oblique muscles of the orbit.

THE KINEMATICS OF JOINTS

Intra-articular kinematics or *arthrokinematics* has to do with the movement of one articular surface upon another. If differs from osteokinematics in two respects: sellar surfaces have to be considered as well as the ovoid type, and *rolling* occurs as well as slide and spin.

5.1 Articular surfaces always occur in *mating pairs;* these always articulate solely with each other. We shall call them *con-articular surfaces*.

5.1.1 One conarticular surface is called male, the other female, following the terminology of engineers. A convex surface is male, a concave is female. The male surface is always larger than the female in such a pair. Hence the larger of two sellar conarticular pairs is also called male, the smaller being called female.

5.2.2. Conarticular surfaces are always curved; there are no truly plane joints, though the term is admissible (by custom!) for those whose surfaces are only slightly curved.

Hence, articular surfaces are *either* ovoid *or* sellar.

5.3. Arthrokinematics is studied in the same way as osteokinematics. We imagine a rodlet to be attached to the moving surface and investigate its motions on the fixed surface.

5.4. Except in one position, characteristic for each joint, the male and female surfaces are incongruous. In what is called the close-packed position the female surface is wholly congruous with the apposed part of the male surface and the two are inseparable by direct traction. The characteristic movements of a bone (4.7) are those towards and away from the close packed position.

5.4.1 All positions of a joint other than the close-packed are called *loose-packed*.

5.5. Articular surfaces can spin and/or slide upon each other. When the joint is ovoid then the kinematics is that already described for the ovoid of motion of a bone. The kinematics of a sellar joint differs from that of an ovoid in two respects: adjunct rotation is never permitted and a clockwise diadochal slide produces an anti-clockwise conjunct rotation of the moving surface. The second difference follows from (1.3) and (3.3).

An example of the second difference is furnished by the left carpometacarpal joint of the thumb. First bring the thumb into full radial deviation and then into full abduction (away from the palm) by the shortest routes: The thumb will be found to have rotated medially—that is, anti-clockwise. But to accomplish this diadochal motion of radial deviation and abduction the articular surface of the metacarpal bone had first to slide medially and then forwards (palmwards) on the trapezium—a clockwise diadochal slide. This illustrates the general theorem.

5.6. *Roll* is of two kinds: male roll and female roll. In male roll a convexity rolls upon a concavity; in female roll a concavity rolls upon a convexity.

5.6.1. Roll and slide are always found together, although they are not always found in equal proportion.

5.6.2. A male roll *per se* would move the surface in the direction opposite to that in which slide actually takes place; a female roll *per se* would move the surface in the same direction as that in which slide actually takes place.

5.7. The general effect of roll and slide is the same: each rotates the axis of the bone through an angle which is of the same sense (fig. A.7 a, b). Thus roll and slide reinforce the effect of each other, as shown in fig. A.7 c.

5.8. Female roll is merely the counterpart of male roll. It has, however, a special interest in connection with the theory of articular lubrication. Imagine a vertical section cut through a female surface (fig. A.8). Label one end *t* (for "tail") and the

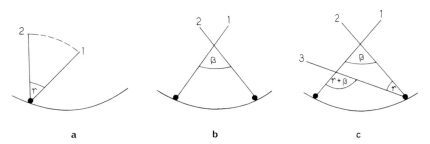

Fig. A.7. The effects of rolling (a), sliding (b) and combined rolling and sliding (c) upon the axis of a bone moving upon an articular surface. The letters indicate angles; the numbers indicate successive positions of the axis.

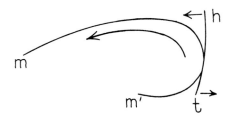

Fig. A.8. To illustrate rolling of a female surface upon a male.

other end h (for "head"). Let the female surface slide on the male in the direction t-h. Because is also rolls on the male surface the female surface will continually move away from the male at the tail-end and approach it at the head-end. Hence the leading (headward) part of the female surface will continually approach the male surface as it slides over the male. This relationship of a moving to a fixed surface is a help to the formation of a lubricant film (pressure-film) between the two surfaces in the neighbourhood of the instantaneous load-bearing part of the conarticular pair. The lubricant is, of course, the synovial fluid. The same phenomenon occurs when a male surface rolls and slides on a female.*

5.8.1. The combination of roll with slide has a further bio-

---

* For a review of lubrication in synovial joints and a bibliography of recent work see MacConaill (1966).

mechanical advantage. Because of the roll not one and the same point but a succession of points of the moving surface comes near a succession of points on the female surface. This is clearly a help towards preventing continuous stress being applied to one area of the articular cartilage with the consequent liability to attrition therefrom. It is significant that senile attrition of articular cartilage is most often found in the regions that come into close contact in close-pack, in which position rolling is virtually impossible.

5.9. The hip and shoulder joints are of a special kind in that the articular surfaces of the femur and humerus, respectively, lie to one side of the axis of the shaft of their respective bones. This is illustrated for the femur in fig. A.9. It follows that what are called flexion and extension of the femur are not due to swings but to *spins* of its neck upon the acetabulum, the same

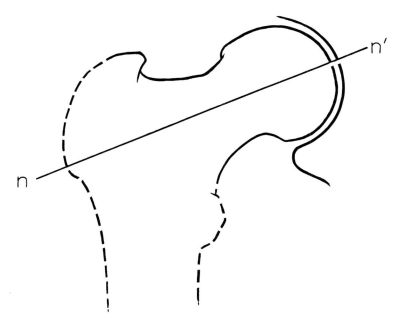

Fig. A.9. To show that flexion and extension of a femur are really spins.

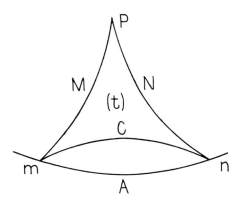

Fig. A.10. To illustrate theorem (5.10).

being true *mutatis mutandis* for the corresponding movements of humerus upon the glenoid cavity.

5.10. Finally, it is to be noted that sellar surfaces are more fitted than ovoid for bringing about the conjunct rotation that accompanies an arcuate slide.

Proof: On any surface draw an arc mAn, as shown in fig. A.10. Draw the corresponding chord mCn. Then draw two intersecting chords mMp and nNp, each at right angles to A. Let the internal angle between M and N (at p) be a. Then the sum of the internal angles of the trigone (M, A, N) will be $(\pi + a)$, and that of the internal angles of the triangle (M, C, N) will be $(\pi + r)$ where r is the residual of the triangle. Then s the sum of the two angles subtended by A on C, is given by:

$$s = (\pi + a) - (\pi + r) = (a - r).$$

Now s is the conjunct rotation due to a slide along the arc A. On a flat surface r is zero and $s = a$, as is well known. On an ovoid surface r is positive and therefore s is less than a—it may even be negative! But on a sellar surface r is negative, so that $-r$ is positive; whence s is always greater than a. It is, of course, assumed that the arc A makes non-zero angles with C.

Hence other things being equal, a sellar arc is more "curved" than an ovoid arc and will give more conjunct rotation than the ovoid arc. The "other things" are the angle a and the length of the arc A in each case. The matter could be dealt with more fully but space does not permit.

REFERENCES

Barnett, C. H., Davies, D. V. and MacConaill, M. A. (1961) *Synovial Joints*. Longmans, London.

MacConaill, M. A. (1946) Studies in the mechanics of synovial joints II. *Irish J. Med. Sci.* 6th series, 223–235.

MacConaill, M. A. (1953) The movements of bones and joints V, *J. Bone Jt. Surg.*, *35B*, 290–297.

MacConaill, M. A. (1964) Joint movements, *Physiotherapy*, November, 359–367.

MacConaill, M. A. (1966) Some ergonomic aspects of articular mechanics. In *Studies on the Anatomy and Function of Bone and Joints*. Ed. by F. Gaynor Evans. Springer-Verlag, Berlin, Heidelberg, New York.

MacConaill, M. A. (1966) The synovial fluid, *Lab. Pract.*, *15*, No. 1 (June).

Theory of Arcuvial Myokinematics
By M. A. MacConaill

This appendix presupposes that Chapter 6 has been read up to the point at which the Appendix is relevant (p. 117). Consequently, symbols used in that chapter will not be defined again; and the diagrams used in it will not be repeated here.

Taken in order, the topics treated of are: the separability of variables, the changes in myonemic length, the kinematics of flexor and/or abductor myonemes, and that of extensor and/or adductor myonemes. Finally, spurt and shunt muscles are considered.

Separability of Variables

Full contraction of an arcuvial myoneme will have associated with it a spin of magnitude R and a swing of magnitude A. In the equations to be found both angles are measured in radians.

Even when two variables change in magnitude together, as do R and A in arcuate motions, mathematical physics allows us to treat them as if one occurred before the other. Thus we can determine the myokinematics of any arcuvial myoneme with respect to R before that with respect to A.

Similarly, the length of a myoneme can be divided into two parts; one of them attached to the moving bone, the other being the remaining part. This is because the amount of partial contraction of a myoneme is independent of the sites of its contracting myonemes. So the separation of a myoneme's length into a spin-fraction and a swing-fraction does not imply that the myoneme has two such separate functional parts.

Changes in Arcuvial Myonemic Length

Let a fully stretched myoneme of length s be one of a set that can both spin a bone through an angle R and swing it through an angle A. Then the spin R can be associated with a contraction of s to a length y; and the swing A will then be associated with the total contraction of s to its smallest possible length z. The reader should refer to Fig. B, and to Chapter 6 in connection with the changes of s to y and of y to z.

The initial length s can be divided into a *gyrovial* part $2Rar$ and the remainder. Here a is an undetermined multiplier of Rr; it is always less, usually much less than $s/2$, but its exact value is not necessary for our present purposes. We have, then:

$$(1.1) \quad s = Rar + (s\text{-}Rar) \quad (\text{Fig. B, } a)$$

We now define two further symbols, ρ and RF:

$$(1.2.1) \quad \rho = Rar$$

$(1.2.2)$ RF = the product of R and any expression(s) that contain ar; but not ρ considered by itself.

The total spin R is accompanied by a change of 2ρ to ρ, and of s to y. Hence

$$(1.3) \quad y = s\text{-}\rho \quad (\text{Fig. B, b})$$

It follows that y is the wholly chordovial part of s, whose gyrovial function is exhausted (by the separation principle). Further, the same principle permits us to associate t, the myoneme's proportion of tendon, to y. The equations to be found for A could also be used as equations for R (in terms of A) and then the part of t in determining R can be assessed. In any case, t is taken full account of in the equation for the change from s to z.

The now fully chordovial myoneme has a "virtual insertion" at the point where it leaves the moving bone to pass to its origin. It passes over an axis of swing and the ·distances from this axis to the virtual insertion and to the myoneme's origin are denoted by q and c, respectively, as with chordovial muscles generally (Fig. B, c and Chapter 6).

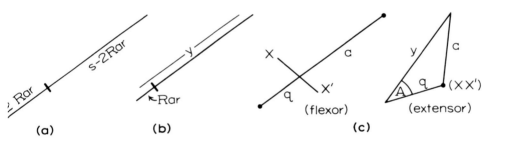

Fig. B. (a) Uncontracted (fully stretched) arcuvial myoneme of length s. (b) Length of same (y) consequent upon spin of bone through total angle R. Division of y by axis of swing XX' (flexor myoneme); and relation of y to lengths c and q (extensor myoneme), as explained in Chapter 6. Further details in text.

Equations for flexor swing apply also to abductor swing; ·and those for extensor swing apply also to adductor swing. This is because in the latter two cases the bone has already been swung through a total angle A, and the myonemes involved bring the swing back to $0°$.

Flexor and/or Abductor Myonemes

$$(2.1) \quad s = y + \rho \quad \text{from (1.2)}$$

$$(2.1.1) \quad y = c + q$$

$$(2.2) \quad z = s(1+t)/2 = (c+q+\rho)(1+t)/2$$

$$(2.2.1) \quad z^2 = \frac{(c+q)^2 (1+t)^2}{4} + RF$$

$$(2.3) \quad z^2 = (c+q)^2 - 4cq \sin^2 A/2 \quad \text{(by Chapter 6)}$$

By equating the above two values of z^2 we find:

$$(2.4) \quad \sin^2 A/2 = \frac{(c+q)^2 (3+t)(1-t)}{16cq} - \frac{RF}{16cq}$$

By putting (2.4) in terms of $p(=c/q)$ we find:

$$(2.5) \quad \sin^2 A/2 = \frac{(p+t)^2 (3+t)(1-t)}{16p} - \frac{R}{16p} F$$

When $R = 0$ then $\sin^2 A/2 = \sin^2 A'/2$, where A is the total swing corresponding to a fully chordovial myoneme. Hence we can write:

$$(2.6) \quad \sin^2 A/2 = \sin^2 A'/2 - \frac{R}{16p}(F)$$

That is, as $R/16p$ becomes smaller so does A become nearer to A', its "fully chordovial" value.

Extensor and/or Adductor Myonemes

In these cases $\sin^2 A/2$ is found by equating the two possible values of y^2 instead of those of z^2.

$$(3.1) \quad z = (c-q) \quad \text{(by Chapter 6)}$$

$$(3.2) \quad s = 2z/(1+t) = 2(c-q)/(1+t)$$

$$(3.3) \quad y = s- \quad = \frac{2(c-q)}{(1+t)} - p$$

$$(3.3.1) \quad y^2 = \frac{4(c-q)^2}{(1+t)^2} - RF$$

$$(3.4) \quad y^2 = (c-q)^2 + 4\,cq\,\sin^2 A/2 \quad \text{(by Chapter 6)}$$

By equating (3.3.1) and (3.2) we find:

$$(3.5) \quad \sin^2 A/2 = \frac{(c-q)^2\,(3+t)\,(1-t)}{4cq(1+t)^2} - \frac{RF}{4cq}$$

Putting (3.5) in terms of p:

$$(3.6) \quad \sin^2 A/2 = \frac{(p-1)^2\,(3+t)\,(1-t)}{4p(1+t)^2} - \frac{R}{4p}(F)$$

$$(3.7) \quad \sin^2 A/2 = \sin^2 A'/2 - \frac{R}{4p}\ (F)$$

where A' is the value of A appropriate to a fully chordovial myoneme (Chapter 6).

Application to Muscles

The equations for $\sin^2 A/2$ obtained above can be applied to the active parts of muscles by the use of the equivalent myonemes of such parts, as described in Chapter 6.

'Spurt' and 'Shunt' Types of Arcuvial Muscles

In Chapter 7 myonemes and muscles are divided for kinetic purposes into "spurt types" and "shunt types." In the spurt types $p \geqslant 1$; in the shunt types $p < 1$. But equations (2.6) and (3.7) above show that these types have also a *kinematic* significance if the myonemes (or muscles) are arcuvial.

Excepting the shoulder and radio-humeral joints, the value of R is never greater than 1.6 radians (just over 90°). Hence:

i) For flexor/abductor myonemes $R/16 \leqslant 1/10$;
ii) For extensor/adductor myonemes $R/4 \leqslant 2/5$.

Spurt types. As p increases from 5 upwards, so does $R/16p$ decrease from 1/60 downwards towards 0 (in the limit). Thus, both moderately and markedly *flexor* and/or *abductor* arcuvial muscles of the spurt type will produce a swing that approximates closely, or even very closely, to that produced by a fully chordovial muscle.

On the other hand, we must have $p \geqslant 32$ for arcuvial *extensor* and/or *adductor* muscles to produce a similar approximation to the effect of fully chordovial types. It would seem, then, that the flexor/abductor type is more efficient than the extensor/adductor type for producing swing, given equal values of s and R for the two types. This, however, is in keeping with the fact that the flexor and abductor muscles are those which move the bones from their normal zero positions. Their action stretches their antagonists to such an extent that these must necessarily be fully as effective as those that stretch them.

Shunt types. Since $p \leqslant 1$ for these types then $R/16p$ and $R/4p$ will be greater than for the spurt types; thus, if $p = 2$, then these quantities become 1/5 and 4/5 respectively. This means that, for given s and R, *shunt muscles are less effective for producing swing that spurt muscles*. The flexor and abductor types are again the better for one and the same p; and the remarks made about the functional role of the types in the preceding paragraph apply to shunt types also.

These conclusions are supported by expanding $RF/16p$ and taking $R \leqslant 1.6$; but this need not be done here.

The Generalized Theory of Centripetal Force

By M. A. MacConaill

This appendix has three purposes. First, to derive Newton's law of centripetal force from the simple fact of angular velocity. Secondly, to generalize it by a simple use of differential and integral calculi. Finally, to apply the generalized law to osteokinetics.

Newton's definition of linear momentum is accepted. Force is defined as a vector whose magnitude is the ratio of an energy to a distance. It is assumed that the reader understands simple vector algebra and the theory of physical dimensions.

1. Symbols

(1.1)   *Vectors* are denoted by italic capitals for typographical reasons; thus, A and R.

(1.2)   The magnitude of vectors and of other scalar quantities are denoted by italic small letters, thus a and r.

(1.3)   The signs ($\times$) and ($\cdot$) denote the vector and the scalar multiplication of vectors, respectively; thus $A \times R$ and $R \cdot N$.

2. Definitions

(2.1)   All vectors and magnitudes are instantaneous unless otherwise stated.

(2.2)   Let a particle of mass m be moving around an instantaneous axis at a distance R from it; the sense of R is unimportant but it can be taken as centripetal if desired. R and m have an angular velocity A around the axis. We define:

(2.2.1) $R \cdot A = 0$

that is, R and (the axis of) A are mutually perpendicular.

(2.3)   Because of A and R, the particle will have a tangential velocity V and therefore a linear momentum P. We define:

(2.3.1) $P \cdot A = \text{in } mV \cdot R = A \cdot R = 0$

that is, P, R and (the axis of) A are mutually perpendicular. We have also the scalar equation:

(2.4) $par = pv = mv^2$

3. Newtonian Centripetal Force

(3.1) A exists, then P exists and $P{\times}A$ also exists. Hence we define:

(3.1.1) $N = P{\times}A = -P{\times}\text{-}A$ from which it follows that:

(3.1.2) $P \cdot N = A \cdot N - N \times R = 0$ (by vector algebra),

that is, P and A and N are mutually perpendicular; and N is a radial (or pararadial) vector.

(3.2) $N \cdot R = nr$

   From vector algebra we find:

(3.3) $nr = par = mv^2$ (by 2.4)

(3.4) $n = mv^2/r = 2e/r$

where e is the kinetic energy of the particle at the instant considered.

We now find the nature of N from the physical dimensions of n, denoted by $[n]$.

(3.5) $\qquad [n] = [mv^2/r] = [mra^2] = [ML/T^2]$.

The dimensions ML/T^2 are those of Force, as this term has been universally accepted since Newton's day. Hence, N is to be accepted as a force-vector unless proof to the contrary be provided.

(3.6) $\qquad$ From (3.4) we find at once the partial differential equations

(3.6.1) $\qquad \partial n/\partial e = 2/r$

(3.6.2) $\qquad \partial n/\partial r = -2e/r^2$

This is the inverse-square-law governing n with respect to r, as first stated by Newton in a different way.

(3.6.3) $\qquad n = 0$ and $N = 0$ if either $A = 0$ or $r =$ infinity; in the latter case V is rectilinear as geometry shows.

It has now been shown that all particle-motions, except a limiting set, are necessarily accompanied by a *radial force;* whose magnitude is determined completely by three quantities, namely, the mass of the particle, the instantaneous radius of curvature of the path and the rate of the angular velocity of the particle at the same instant. The part assigned to rectilinear motion by Newton is reversed; it is now taken as a special case of general motion. Consequently, the part assigned to radial force by him is now changed; it may be a consequence, not a cause, of the curvilinear, much more usual, type of motion.

The radial force may be either centripetal or centrifugal. Either form suffices *a priori.* Newton's use of centripetal force in explaining curvilinear motion was a necessary consequence of his first postulate (called "law") of motion. This is not a treatise on general mechanics, so the matter will not be pursued here save for one remark. *Radial force, centripetal or the reverse is a consequence of curvature of a path,* even in non-relativistic physics. This is a fundamental fact in osteokinetics.

It has been shown in (3.1.1) that the sense of a radial force is independent of the sense of A. That it is centripetal in osteokinetics will be proved later.

4. The Generalized Newtonian Law

From now onwards only scalar quantities (magnitudes) are necessary to denote forces.

To begin with, equation (3.4) may be looked upon as a particular solution of a purely mathematical equation:

(4.1) $df/dn = 1$; of which the general solution is:

(4.2) $f = n + b$ in which;

(4.2.1) $db/dn = 0$

that is, b is independent of n.

Homogeneity of equation (4.2) requires that the dimensions and nature of b should be the same as those of n. Hence b is the magnitude of a *force;* and can be taken as that of a radial force along the same line of action of the "Newtonian" force n.

If $n = 0$ then $f = b$; that is b stands for a *static force* acting when (say) a particle is at rest. In theory it may be 0 or have a non-zero value. In elementary celestial mechanics, say, of a planet and a satellite removed from all other bodies, it is taken to be 0. This is not always true in biomechanics.

Equation (4.2) is the *Generalized Newtonian Law* of radial force. Systems conforming to it will be called *Newtonic* for brevity if b is not 0.

5. Newtonic Transarticular Force

In osteokinetics and myokinetics the gravicentre of a mobile bone takes the place of a material particle. It is convenient to replace m, the symbol for its mass, by w/g, where w and g have their usual physical meanings.

In Chapter 7 of the text it is shown that the total transarticular force of a mobile bone at rest in the antipendent position is w. If j denotes the transarticular force of such a bone; and if j is constant for any position of a stationary bone: then $j = w$.

When the bone moves it is constrained by its muscles and ligaments to move upon the curved articular surface of its conarticular bone. Hence its motion is curvilinear and this generates an instantaneous radial force n at any chosen point of its path (*i.e.* of the gravicentre path). We then have:

(5.1) $\qquad j = n + b$

If the system be Newtonic b is constant and:

(5.2) $\qquad j = n + w$

It is known that w is centripetal. What about n?

It is also centripetal. If it were not, the value of j when the bone was antipendent would be less than w, being reduced by the amount n. The force j would then be less than the minimum need for safety of the joint (Chapter 7). Now the path of a gravicentre relative to the joint at which it moves is monotonic, that is, it has no point of inflexion. Thus the senses of p and a, therefore of n, do not change during the journey along the path in either direction (by 3.1.1). Hence n is always centripetal; and j is also centripetal.

Hence we have:

(5.3) $\qquad j = (n + w) = (w + wv^2/gr) = w(1+v^2/gr)$

(5.3.1) $\qquad j = w (1 + ra^2 / g)$.

Simple experiments, on large joints and small, show that if a be measured in radian/sec, then $a^2 < 10$. Measuring r in cm. and g in cm/sec², we can therefore write:

(5.3.2) $\qquad j = w (1+r/100)$.

Thus the centripetal force will significantly exceed the weight of the moving part only when r exceeds 10 cm and a is rapid.*

---

*Equation (5.3) was first published in MacConaill, M.A. (1957). Studies in the mechanics of synovial joints, V: Motion at one joint. *Ir. J. Med. Sc.* (1957), pp. 99-113. The present appendix is a more rigorous study of the whole matter.

INDEX